Vascular Medicine

Editors

STANISLAV HENKIN
MARK A. CREAGER

CARDIOLOGY CLINICS

www.cardiology.theclinics.com

November 2021 • Volume 39 • Number 4

ELSEVIER

1600 John F. Kennedy Boulevard • Suite 1800 • Philadelphia, Pennsylvania, 19103-2899

http://www.theclinics.com

CARDIOLOGY CLINICS Volume 39, Number 4
November 2021 ISSN 0733-8651, ISBN-13: 978-0-323-83524-4

Editor: Joanna Collett
Developmental Editor: Karen Justine Solomon

Cardiology Clinics (ISSN 0733-8651) is published quarterly by Elsevier Inc., 360 Park Avenue South, New York, NY 10010-1710. Months of issue are February, May, August, and November. Business and Editorial Offices: 1600 John F. Kennedy Blvd., Ste. 1800, Philadelphia, PA 19103-2899. Customer Service Office: 3251 Riverport Lane, Maryland Heights, MO 63043. Periodicals postage paid at New York, NY and additional mailing offices. Subscription prices are $359.00 per year for US individuals, $929.00 per year for US institutions, $100.00 per year for US students and residents, $445.00 per year for Canadian individuals, $962.00 per year for Canadian institutions, $466.00 per year for international individuals, $962.00 per year for international institutions, $100.00 per year for Canadian students/residents and $220.00 per year for international students/residents. To receive student/resident rate, orders must be accompanied by name of affiliated institution, data of term, and the *signature* of program/residency coordinator on institution letterhead. Orders will be billed at individual rate until proof of status is received. Foreign air speed delivery is included in all *Clinics* subscription prices. All prices are subject to change without notice. **POSTMASTER:** Send address changes to *Cardiology Clinics*, Elsevier Health Sciences Division, Subscription Customer Service, 3251 Riverport Lane, Maryland Heights, MO 63043. **Customer Service: 1-800-654-2452 (U.S. and Canada); 314-447-8871 (outside U.S. and Canada). Fax: 314-447-8029. E-mail: journalscustomerservice-usa@elsevier.com (for print support); journalsonlinesupport-usa@elsevier.com (for online support).**

Reprints. For copies of 100 or more, of articles in this publication, please contact the Commercial Reprints Department, Elsevier Inc., 360 Park Avenue South, New York, NY 10010-1710. Tel.: 212-633-3874; Fax: 212-633-3820; E-mail: reprints@elsevier.com.

Cardiology Clinics is also published in Spanish by McGraw-Hill Interamericana Editores S. A., P.O. Box 5-237, 06500, Mexico D. F., Mexico; in Portuguese by Reichmann and Alfonso Editores Rio de Janeiro, Brazil; and in Greek by Dimitrios P. Lagos, 8 Pondon Street, GR115-28 Ilissia, Greece.

Cardiology Clinics is covered in *MEDLINE/PubMed (Index Medicus), Excerpta Medica, The Cumulative Index to Nursing and Allied Health Literature* (CINAHL).

Contributors

ANA I. CASANEGRA, MD, MS
Associate Professor of Medicine, Vascular
Medicine Division, Cardiovascular
Department, Gonda Vascular Center, Mayo
Clinic, Rochester, Minnesota

RANDALL R. DEMARTINO, MD, MS
Division of Vascular and Endovascular Surgery,
Mayo Clinic, Rochester, Minnesota

YOUNG ERBEN, MD
Department of Vascular Surgery, Mayo Clinic,
Jacksonville, Florida

CAMILA FRANCO-MESA, MD
Department of Vascular Surgery, Mayo Clinic,
Jacksonville, Florida

ERI FUKAYA, MD, PhD
Division of Vascular Surgery, Vascular
Medicine Section, Stanford University,
Stanford, California

J. ANTONIO GUTIERREZ, MD, MHS
Division of Cardiology, Department of
Medicine, Duke University Health System,
Durham, North Carolina

STANISLAV HENKIN, MD, MPH
Director, Vascular Medicine Program,
Dartmouth-Hitchcock Medical Center, Assistant
Professor of Medicine, Dartmouth Geisel School
of Medicine, Lebanon, New Hampshire

CONNIE N. HESS, MD, MHS
Division of Cardiology, University of Colorado,
School of Medicine, Section of Vascular Medicine,
CPC Clinical Research, Aurora, Colorado

TARA A. HOLDER, MD
Division of Cardiovascular Medicine,
Vanderbilt University Medical Center,
Nashville, Tennessee

ANNA K. KRAWISZ, MD
Cardiovascular Medicine Fellow, Department
of Medicine, Richard A. and Susan F. Smith
Center for Outcomes Research in Cardiology,
Division of Cardiology, Department of
Medicine, Beth Israel Deaconess Medical
Center, Harvard Medical School, Boston,
Massachusetts

SHANTUM MISRA, MD
Department of Medicine, Dartmouth-
Hitchcock Medical Center, Lebanon, New
Hampshire

ABBY M. PRIBISH, MD
Department of Medicine, Division of ADM-
Housestaff, Beth Israel Deaconess Medical
Center, Harvard Medical School, Boston,
Massachusetts

T. BRETT REECE, MD
Division of Cardiovascular Surgery, University
of Colorado, School of Medicine, Aurora,
Colorado

R. KEVIN ROGERS, MD, MSc
Division of Cardiology, University of Colorado,
School of Medicine, Section of Vascular
Medicine, Aurora, Colorado

ALEC A. SCHMAIER, MD, PhD
Division of Cardiology, Department of
Medicine, Beth Israel Deaconess Medical
Center, Harvard Medical School, Boston,
Massachusetts

ERIC A. SECEMSKY, MD, MSc
Assistant Professor, Department of
Medicine, Investigator, Richard A. and Susan
F. Smith Center for Outcomes Research in
Cardiology, Director of Vascular Intervention,
Assistant Professor of Medicine, Harvard
Medical School, Division of Cardiology,
Department of Medicine, Beth Israel
Deaconess Medical Center, Boston,
Massachusetts

INDRANI SEN, MD
Division of Vascular and Endovascular Surgery,
Mayo Clinic, Rochester, Minnesota

ETHAN M. SENSER, MD
Heart and Vascular Center, Dartmouth-
Hitchcock Medical Center, Lebanon, New
Hampshire

SWAPNA SHARMA, MD, MS
The Elliot Hospital, Manchester, New
Hampshire

ROGER F. SHEPHERD, MB BCh
Associate Professor of Medicine, Vascular
Medicine Division, Cardiovascular
Department, Gonda Vascular Center, Mayo
Clinic, Rochester, Minnesota

MICHAEL N. YOUNG, MD
Assistant Professor of Medicine, Heart and
Vascular Center, Dartmouth-Hitchcock
Medical Center, Lebanon, New Hampshire

Contents

> Peripheral artery disease is a highly morbid yet undertreated atherosclerotic disease. The cornerstones of peripheral artery disease therapy consist of smoking cessation, lipid-lowering therapy, and hypertension treatment. More recently, clinical trials have demonstrated that novel antiplatelet and antithrombotic therapies reduce the risk of both cardiovascular and limb events in this patient population. In this review, we highlight the components of optimal medical therapy of peripheral artery disease and the evidence base for these therapies.

> Chronic limb-threatening ischemia requires aggressive risk factor management and a thoughtful approach to the complex decision of best strategy for revascularization. Patients often have multilevel disease amenable to endovascular, open surgical, or hybrid approaches. Limited high-quality evidence is available to support a specific strategy; randomized trials are ongoing. Acute limb ischemia is associated with a high risk of limb loss and mortality. Catheter-directed thrombolysis is mainstay of therapy in patients with marginally threatened limbs, whereas those immediately threatened with motor deficits require more rapid restoration of flow with open or endovascular techniques that can establish flow in single setting.

 Video content accompanies this article at http://www.cardiology.theclinics.com.

> Acute aortic syndromes, classified into aortic dissection, intramural hematoma, and penetrating aortic ulcer, are associated with high early mortality for which early diagnosis and management are crucial to optimize outcomes. Patients often present with nonspecific clinical symptoms and signs; therefore, it is important for providers to maintain a high index of suspicion for acute aortic syndromes. Electrocardiogram-gated computed tomographic angiography of the chest, abdomen, and pelvis is currently the most practical imaging modality for diagnosis and identification of complications. Evolution in surgical techniques and the development of aortic endografts have improved patient outcomes, but randomized trials are still needed.

> Thoracic aortic aneurysms are common. Most thoracic aortic aneurysms are degenerative. However, some are associated with connective tissue disorders, bicuspid

aortic valves, or familial/genetic predisposition. Most are asymptomatic, discovered incidentally on imaging. Aortic diameter is the best predictor of the natural history and risk of complications. Treating hypertension and smoking cessation can slow their growth. Surveillance imaging and referral for prophylactic aortic repair based on absolute aneurysm diameter is the primary means to decrease mortality from thoracic aortic aneurysm. We provide a practical evidence-based summary of the pathophysiology, risk factors, associated genetic syndromes, and clinical management of thoracic aortic aneurysms.

Abdominal aortic aneurysms account for nearly 9000 deaths annually, with ruptured abdominal aortic aneurysms being the thirteenth leading cause of death in the United States. Abdominal aortic aneurysms can be detected by screening, but a majority are detected incidentally. Visceral artery aneurysms are often discovered incidentally, and treatment is guided by symptoms, etiology, and size. A timely diagnosis and referral to a vascular specialist are essential for timely open or endovascular repair and to ensure successful patient outcomes.

Renal artery stenosis is caused by atherosclerosis and fibromuscular dysplasia and is associated with ischemic nephropathy, renovascular hypertension, and accelerated cardiovascular disease. Routine screening for renal artery stenosis is not recommended but is reasonable in patients who have rapid onset of hypertension, resistant hypertension, progressive renal insufficiency, recurrent pulmonary edema, or repeat admissions for heart failure. Acute mesenteric ischemia is caused by arterial embolism or thrombosis, mesenteric venous thrombosis, or nonocclusive mesenteric ischemia, whereas chronic mesenteric ischemia is most often caused by arterial obstruction. This article reviews the epidemiology, pathophysiology, diagnosis, and management of these two conditions.

Stroke is the fifth leading cause of death in the United States and is a leading cause of disability. Extracranial internal carotid artery stenosis is a major cause of ischemic stroke, as it is estimated to cause 8% to 15% of ischemic strokes. It is critical to improve our strategies for stroke prevention and treatment in order to reduce the burden of this disease. Herein, we review approaches for the diagnosis and risk stratification of carotid artery disease as well as interventional strategies for the prevention and treatment of strokes caused by carotid artery disease.

Venous thromboembolism (VTE), encompassing pulmonary embolism (PE) and deep vein thrombosis (DVT), is encountered commonly. Acute PE may present as a high-risk cardiovascular emergency, and acute DVT can cause acute and chronic vascular complications. The goal of this review is to ensure that cardiologists are comfortable managing VTE—including risk stratification, anticoagulation therapy, and familiarity with primary reperfusion therapy. Clinical assessment and determination of degree of right ventricular dysfunction are critical in initial risk stratification of PE and determination of parenteral versus oral anticoagulation therapy. Direct oral anticoagulants have emerged as preferred first-line oral anticoagulation strategy in VTE scenarios.

Chronic venous disease is a worldwide problem associated with significant morbidity and is expected to increase in prevalence as the current population ages. This is a comprehensive review of the anatomy, pathophysiology, genomics, clinical classification, and treatment modalities of chronic venous disease.

Vasospastic disorders are prevalent in the general population and can affect individuals of any age. Primary (or idiopathic) vasospastic disorders often have a benign course; treatment focuses on the control of symptoms. Secondary vasospastic disorders occur owing to an underlying condition and have an increased risk of complications, including tissue loss and digital ulcerations; treatment should focus on the underlying condition. In this review, we discuss the pathophysiology, clinical presentation, diagnosis, and management of vasospastic disorders, including Raynaud syndrome, acrocyanosis, livedo reticularis, and pernio.

CARDIOLOGY CLINICS

SERIES OF RELATED INTEREST

Cardiac Electrophysiology Clinics
Available at: https://www.cardiacep.theclinics.com/
Heart Failure Clinics
Available at: https://www.heartfailure.theclinics.com/
Interventional Cardiology Clinics
Available at: https://www.interventional.theclinics.com/

THE CLINICS ARE AVAILABLE ONLINE!
Access your subscription at:
www.theclinics.com

Preface
Management of Vascular Disorders in Cardiovascular Practice

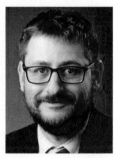 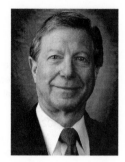

Stanislav Henkin, MD, MPH   Mark A. Creager, MD

Editors

Although cardiovascular disease includes common and possibly life-threatening disorders, such as peripheral artery disease (PAD), venous thromboembolism (VTE), aortic aneurysm, cerebrovascular disease, and others, peripheral vascular diseases are often underdiagnosed and undertreated. Individuals with polyvascular disease (ie, atherosclerosis in multiple arterial beds) are at higher risk of major adverse events and mortality than patients with coronary artery disease or peripheral vascular disease alone. Also, the average annual expenditure is up to 3 times higher for patients with PAD compared with those without PAD.[1] Stroke and VTE are the second and third leading causes of cardiovascular deaths in the United States, respectively.[2] Acute aortic syndrome is associated with significant morbidity and mortality, unless diagnosed and treated in a timely manner; identification and prophylactic treatment of aortic aneurysms may prevent these complications. Up to 15% of Medicare beneficiaries have chronic wounds; almost $1 billion is spent annually on treatment of venous ulcers in the United States.[3] Finally, although rarely life-threatening, vasospastic disorders are associated with decreased quality of life, unless diagnosed and treated appropriately. As the population continues to age, the prevalence and cost of these disorders will continue to increase. Thus, cardiovascular physicians need to be well versed in the

Cardiol Clin 39 (2021) ix–x
https://doi.org/10.1016/j.ccl.2021.07.001
0733-8651/21/© 2021 Published by Elsevier Inc.

initial workup and management of peripheral vascular disorders.

The subspecialty field of vascular medicine continues to grow to address the unique challenges of patients with peripheral vascular diseases. Vascular medicine is part of the core cardiovascular training curriculum (COCATS).[4] In addition, the recent Advanced Training Statement on Vascular Medicine defines the necessary training to become an expert in vascular medicine.[5]

The current issue of *Cardiology Clinics* highlights common vascular disorders encountered in the cardiovascular clinic, authored by experts in cardiovascular medicine and surgery. Understanding cause, pathophysiology, natural history, and management of these diseases is key to reducing adverse events associated with PAD; VTE and venous insufficiency; carotid disease; aortic and visceral artery aneurysms and dissection; renovascular and mesenteric vascular disease; and vasospastic disorders. These topics are important to primary care physicians, cardiologists, cardiovascular surgeons, neurologists, rheumatologists, nephrologists, hematologists, and trainees in these fields interested in multidisciplinary care of patients with peripheral vascular disorders.

Stanislav Henkin, MD, MPH
Heart and Vascular Center
Dartmouth-Hitchcock Medical Center
1 Medical Center Drive
Lebanon, NH 03756, USA

Mark A. Creager, MD
Heart and Vascular Center
Dartmouth-Hitchcock Medical Center
1 Medical Center Drive
Lebanon, NH 03756, USA

E-mail addresses:
stanislav.henkin@hitchcock.org (S. Henkin)
Mark.A.Creager@hitchcock.org (M.A. Creager)

REFERENCES

1. Scully RE, Arnaoutakis DJ, DeBord Smith A, et al. Estimated annual health care expenditures in individuals with peripheral arterial disease. J Vasc Surg 2018;67(2):558–67. https://doi.org/10.1016/j.jvs.2017.06.102.

2. Virani SS, Alonso A, Aparicio HJ, et al. Heart disease and stroke statistics—2021 update: a report from the American Heart Association. Circulation 2021;143(8):e254–743. https://doi.org/10.1161/CIR.0000000000000950.

3. Nussbaum SR, Carter MJ, Fife CE, et al. An economic evaluation of the impact, cost, and medicare policy implications of chronic nonhealing wounds. Value Health 2018;21(1):27–32. https://doi.org/10.1016/j.jval.2017.07.007.

4. Creager MA, Gornik HL, Gray BH, et al. COCATS 4 task force 9: training in vascular medicine. J Am Coll Cardiol 2015;65(17):1832–43. https://doi.org/10.1016/j.jacc.2015.03.025.

5. Creager MA, Hamburg NM, Calligaro KD, et al. 2021 ACC/AHA/SVM/ACP advanced training statement on vascular medicine (revision of the 2004 ACC/ACP/SCAI/SVMB/SVS clinical competence statement on vascular medicine and catheter-based peripheral vascular interventions). Circ Cardiovasc Interv 2021;14(2):e000079. https://doi.org/10.1161/HCV.0000000000000079.

Medical Management of Peripheral Artery Disease

Tara A. Holder, MD[a], J. Antonio Gutierrez, MD, MHS[b], Aaron W. Aday, MD, MSc[a,c,*]

KEYWORDS

- Peripheral artery disease • Statins • Smoking cessation • Antiplatelet therapy
- Antithrombotic therapy

KEY POINTS

- Peripheral artery disease is a progressive atherosclerotic disease that remains underappreciated and poorly optimized.
- The target low-density lipoprotein cholesterol for this patient population is <70 mg/dL (1.8 mmol/L).
- Lipid-lowering therapy improves both cardiovascular and limb outcomes in peripheral artery disease.
- Angiotensin-converting enzyme inhibitors and aldosterone receptor antagonists remain the only antihypertensive therapies with a mortality benefit in peripheral artery disease.
- Aspirin plus low-dose rivaroxaban (2.5 mg twice daily) should be considered in high-risk patients with peripheral artery disease, such as those with a prior history of lower extremity revascularization or with atherosclerosis in other vascular territories.

INTRODUCTION

Lower extremity peripheral artery disease (PAD) is a malignant form of atherosclerosis associated with a heightened risk of cardiovascular morbidity and mortality.[1] Many patients with PAD have additional comorbidities, such as diabetes mellitus or atherosclerosis in additional vascular beds, further amplifying this risk.[2] Much of the medical management of PAD overlaps with secondary prevention of coronary artery disease (CAD) and cerebrovascular disease. In the last 2 decades, greater attention to PAD has led to the development of novel therapies that decrease adverse cardiovascular and limb events in this patient population. This review focuses on the components of optimal medical management of patients with PAD.

SMOKING CESSATION

Tobacco use is strongly associated with cardiovascular disease and remains an important risk factor for the development and progression of PAD.[3] Ongoing smoking is associated with an increased risk of chronic limb-threatening ischemia (CLTI), need for revascularization and amputation, and major adverse cardiovascular events (MACE).[4,5] Observational data from patients with PAD who successfully stop smoking demonstrate improved outcomes,[6] making smoking cessation a primary target for clinicians.

Funding: This work was supported by NIH K23 HL151871 (Dr Aday).
[a] Division of Cardiovascular Medicine, Vanderbilt University Medical Center, 2220 Pierce Avenue, 383 PRB, Nashville, TN 37232-0021, USA; [b] Division of Cardiology, Department of Medicine, Duke University Medical Center, DUMC 3330, Durham, NC 27710, USA; [c] Vanderbilt Translational and Clinical Cardiovascular Research Center, Division of Cardiovascular Medicine, Vanderbilt University Medical Center, Nashville, TN, USA
* Corresponding author. Vanderbilt University Medical Center, 2525 West End Avenue Suite 300, Nashville, TN 37203.
E-mail address: aaron.w.aday@vumc.org
Twitter: @TaraHolder17 (T.A.H.); @JAGutierrezMD (J.A.G.); @AaronAdayMD (A.W.A.)

Cardiol Clin 39 (2021) 471–482
https://doi.org/10.1016/j.ccl.2021.06.001

Current smoking cessation strategies consist of both counseling and pharmacologic intervention with nicotine replacement therapy (NRT), bupropion, or varenicline. A previous study randomizing patients with PAD to either intensive counseling intervention or minimal intervention showed that patients in the intensive intervention group were more likely to achieve smoking abstinence at 6 months compared with the minimal intervention group (21.3% vs 6.8%, P = .023).[7] However, long-term abstinence often requires medical therapy (Table 1).

Bupropion is a norepinephrine and dopamine reuptake inhibitor. When used alone or in addition to nicotine replacement, bupropion leads to higher rates of smoking cessation at 12 months compared with placebo or NRT alone.[8] Varenicline is a partial agonist of α-4 and β-2 nicotinic acetylcholine receptors and remains the most effective smoking cessation aid. Randomized controlled trial data demonstrate that varenicline is more effective than placebo (odds ratio [OR], 3.61; 95% confidence interval [CI], 3.07–4.24), bupropion (OR, 1.68; 95% CI, 1.46–1.93) and nicotine patch (OR, 1.75; 95% CI, 1.52–2.01) at improving 12-week smoking abstinence rates.[9] Importantly, varenicline does not lead to an increase risk of neuropsychiatric side effects.[9]

Recommendations

Current professional guidelines recommend that all patients using tobacco should be advised to quit.[10] For patients that are willing to quit, shared decision-making can be used to determine the best pharmacologic treatment option with either NRT, bupropion, or varenicline.[11] Varenicline, either alone or in combination with NRT, is recommended as the first-line treatment in patients with cardiovascular disease. Based on availability of tobacco cessation programs and patient preference, counseling or group therapy may also be used.[11]

LIPID-LOWERING THERAPY

Dyslipidemia is an important modifiable risk factor in the development of cardiovascular disease and atherosclerosis. Atherogenic dyslipidemia, which is characterized by elevated concentrations of total cholesterol and low levels of high-density lipoprotein cholesterol, is a strong risk factor for PAD development.[12] In contrast with CAD, data demonstrating a link between low-density lipoprotein cholesterol (LDL-C) and incident PAD are sparse. Nonetheless, recent studies have shown a consistent benefit in lipid reduction to decrease MACE, as well as limb outcomes in patients with PAD.

Statin Therapy

Although many patients with PAD participated in the landmark statin trials, PAD-specific outcome data are limited. In the Heart Protection Study, 20,536 high-risk patients with stable vascular disease, of whom 6748 had PAD, were randomized to either simvastatin or placebo. Simvastatin not only decreased the risk of all-cause mortality, but also led to a 16% relative decrease in the rate of first peripheral vascular event, irrespective of baseline LDL-C levels.[13] There was no decrease in amputations with simvastatin compared with placebo.

Observational studies have helped solidify the role of statins in improving PAD outcomes. The international Reduction of Atherothrombosis for Continued Health Registry, which included 5861 patients with symptomatic PAD, demonstrated that statin use was associated with a reduction in adverse limb events compared with those not taking statins (hazard ratio [HR] 0.82; 95% CI, 0.72–0.92, P = .01).[14] Among 155,647 patients with newly diagnosed PAD in the Veterans Affairs health system, statins, particularly high-intensity statin therapy, significantly decreased the rates of lower extremity amputation compared with antiplatelet therapy alone (HR, 0.67; 95% CI, 0.61–0.74).[15]

Ezetimibe

The Improved Reduction of Outcomes: Vytorin Efficacy International Trial (n = 18,144) examined the addition of ezetimibe, which inhibits absorption of cholesterol from the intestine, to simvastatin in patients with recent acute coronary syndrome. Within the trial, 1005 participants had a prior history of PAD. The addition of ezetimibe further decreased LDL-C by approximately 24% along with a reduction in MACE (HR, 0.94; 95% CI, 0.89–0.99; P = .016).[16] Limb events were not reported in this study.

PCSK9 inhibition

More recently, inhibitors of protein convertase subtilisin kexin type 9 (PCSK9) have been shown to not only decrease LDL-C concentrations in patients on statin therapy, but also to decrease the risk cardiovascular and limb events. The Further Cardiovascular Outcomes Research with PCSK9 Inhibition in Subjects with Elevated Risk trial randomized 27,564 patients with known atherosclerotic disease already on a statin to either evolocumab, a PCSK9 inhibitor, or placebo. In a subgroup analysis of 3642 patients with PAD, evolocumab led to a greater decrease in MACE (HR, 0.73; 95% CI, 0.59–0.91; P = .0040).[17] Although evolocumab led to a decrease in major adverse

Table 1
Pharmacologic treatment options for smoking cessation

Pharmaceutical	Dosing Strengths	Dosing	OTC	Evidence	Precautions	Side Effects	Dose Adjustments
Short-acting agents							
Nicotine gum	2 mg[a] 4 mg[b]	1 pc, q1–2 h × 6 wk 1 pc, q2–4 h × 3 wk 1 pc, q4–8 h × 3 wk Max: 24 pc/d	Yes	RCT[53]	None	Jaw pain, sleep disturbance, vivid dreams, oral irritation	None[c]
Nicotine lozenge	2 mg[a] 4 mg[b]	1 pc, q1–2 h × 6 wk 1 pc, q2–4 h × 3 wk 1 pc, q4–8 h × 3 wk Max: 20 pc/d	Yes	RCT[53]	None	Jaw pain, sleep disturbance, vivid dreams, oral irritation	None[c]
Nicotine inhaler	10 mg/cartridge	6–16 cartridges/d × 3–6 wk Reduce dose × 6–12 wk Max: 16 cartridges/d	No	RCT[54,55]	None	Headache, oral irritation, nasal discomfort, dyspepsia	None[c]
Nicotine intranasal spray	10 mg/mL (1 spray = 0.5 mg) (2 spray = 1 dose) (1 spray/nostril)	1–2 dose/h (1 spray/nostril) No more than 5 doses (10 sprays) per hour Max: 40 mg/d (80 spray) or 3 mo treatment	No	ND	None	Headache, oral irritation, nasal discomfort, dyspepsia	None[c]
Long-acting agents							
Nicotine patch	14 mg (≤10 cig/d) 21 mg (>10 cig/d)	14 mg/d × 6 wk 7 mg/d × 2 wk 21 mg/d × 6 wk 14 mg/d × 2 wk 7 mg/d × 2 wk	No	RCT[56]	None	Local skin irritation, headaches, insomnia	None[c]
Bupropion	150 mg	150 mg/d × 3 d followed by 150 mg bid × 7–12 wk Max: 300 mg/d	No	RCT[8]	Seizure disorder, SI, use of MAOIs, simultaneous cessation of EtOH or Benzos	Insomnia, agitation, constipation	None[c]

(continued on next page)

Table 1
(continued)

Pharmaceutical	Dosing Strengths	Dosing	OTC	Evidence	Precautions	Side Effects	Dose Adjustments
Varenicline	0.5 mg	0.5 mg/d × 3 d 0.5 mg bid × 4–7 d 1.0 mg bid × 11 wk Max: 2.0 mg/d	No	RCT[9]	*Black box warning for neuropsychiatric events removed in 2016[57]	Nausea, vivid dreams	CrCl <30 mL/min Initial: 0.5 mg/d Max: 0.5 mg bid

Abbreviations: benzos, benzodiazepines; bid, twice daily; cig, cigarettes; CrCl, creatinine clearance; EtOH, alcohol; MAOi, monoamine oxidase inhibitors; ND, no data; OTC, over-the-counter; pc, piece; RCT, randomized controlled trial; SI, suicidal ideation.

Consider adjustments in moderate to severe renal/hepatic impairment.

a Smoke first cigarette after 30 minutes of waking.

b Smoke first cigarette within 30 minutes of waking.

c None provided on manufacturer labeling.

limb events in the overall study population, this decrease did not reach statistical significance in the PAD subgroup. In the ODYSSEY Outcomes trial, treatment with the PCSK9 inhibitor alirocumab did demonstrate a statistically significant reduction in a composite of CLTI, lower extremity amputation, or revascularization (HR, 0.69; 95% CI, 0.54–0.89; $P = .004$).[18]

Recommendations

The US guidelines recommend that all patients with PAD be treated with high-intensity statin therapy for a goal LDL-C decrease of 50% or greater,[19] whereas the European guidelines recommend a target LDL-C of less than 70 mg/dL.[20] High-intensity statin options include atorvastatin 40 to 80 mg/d or rosuvastatin 20 to 40 mg/d. In patients with PAD who do not achieve their target LDL-C on statin therapy alone, additional lipid-lowering therapy with ezetimibe or a PCSK9 inhibitor should be used.[19]

HYPERTENSION

Hypertension is associated with a doubling in the risk of death from stroke, heart disease, or other vascular disease.[21] Current professional guidelines recommend a target blood pressure less than 130/80 mm Hg in patients with cardiovascular disease, including PAD.[22] There remain few studies guiding target blood pressure or specific hypertensive therapeutic choices in patients with PAD. The subgroup analysis of the Appropriate Blood Pressure Control in Diabetes study examined patients with diabetes and PAD (ankle-brachial index [ABI] of <0.90) who were randomized to moderate blood pressure control (placebo, no intended change in diastolic blood pressure) or intensive blood pressure control (enalapril or nisoldipine, target decrease in diastolic blood pressure of 10 mm Hg). The intensive treatment group had a larger reduction in cardiovascular events compared with moderate treatment.[23] The Heart Outcomes Prevention Evaluation trial (n = 4051) randomized patients with vascular disease or diabetes, of whom 44% had PAD, to ramipril 10 mg/d or placebo. Overall, ramipril significantly decreased the risk of MACE in the PAD subgroup.[24] Other clinical trials have found similar reductions in MACE for patients with PAD treated with either angiotensin-converting enzyme inhibitors or angiotensin receptor blockers.[25,26]

There has long been concern that intensive blood pressure control may contribute to adverse limb outcomes in patients with PAD owing to worsened limb perfusion. Among 2699 participants with PAD in the INternational VErapamil-SR/Trandolapril Study, there was a J-shaped relationship between systolic blood pressure and a composite of all-cause death, myocardial infarction, or stroke.[27] Excess risk occurred with a systolic blood pressure of less than 135 mm Hg, suggesting that these patients might require different blood pressure targets. Similarly, the Antihypertensive and Lipid-Lowering Treatment to Prevent Heart Attack Trial (n = 33,357) found that patients with a systolic blood pressure of less than 120 mm Hg or greater than 160 mm Hg were at greater risk of PAD-related outcomes.[28] In contrast, recent data from the Examining the Use of Ticagrelor in Peripheral Artery Disease (EUCLID) trial showed that every 10 mm Hg decrease in systolic blood pressure of 125 mm Hg or less was associated with an increased risk of MACE (HR, 1.19; 95% CI, 1.09–1.31; $P<.001$) but no increased risk of adverse limb events (HR, 1.02%; 95%, 0.84–1.23; $P = .824$).[29] Additional work is needed to better understand the link between PAD and hypertension.

Recommendations

In patients with PAD, the American College of Cardiology/American Heart Association PAD guidelines recommend targeting a blood pressure of less than 130/80 mm Hg.[10] Angiotensin-converting enzyme inhibitors of angiotensin receptor blockers are the only antihypertensive medications with a mortality benefit in the PAD population and should remain the first-line therapies in this population. Current data suggest that intensive blood pressure control in patients with PAD, particularly those with more advanced PAD, may worsen limb symptoms, thus necessitating a more liberal target in select groups. PAD-specific blood pressure targets have yet to be defined.

ANTIPLATELET AND ANTITHROMBOTIC THERAPY
Antiplatelet Therapy

Antiplatelet and antithrombotic therapy remain key components of primary and secondary prevention of cardiovascular disease. Although antiplatelet therapy has historically been used to treat a wide range of atherosclerotic diseases, data supporting the use of these drugs in PAD, particularly in terms of decreasing adverse limb outcomes, are inconsistent. More recently, a combination of antiplatelet and antithrombotic therapy has shown significant benefits among patients with PAD, and these drug regimens represent a paradigm shift in PAD management (**Table 2**).

Aspirin

Aspirin is a cyclooxygenase-1 inhibitor that inhibits the effect of thromboxane A2, thus inhibiting platelet aggregation. The ATT Collaboration meta-analysis showed that patients with symptomatic PAD on antiplatelet therapy had a 22% reduction in MACE. Although this analysis used various aspirin doses and other antithrombotic therapies, this marks the earliest clinical evidence supporting antiplatelet therapy in PAD.[30]

More recent studies have shown a less consistent benefit of aspirin therapy. The Prevention of Progression of Arterial Disease and Diabetes trial (n = 1276) assessed the efficacy of aspirin 100 mg versus placebo in patients with diabetes and PAD. The study found no difference between groups in cardiovascular end points (18.2% vs 18.3%), nor was there a difference in lower extremity amputation.[31] The Aspirin for Asymptomatic Atherosclerosis Trial (n = 3350) examined aspirin 100 mg versus placebo in patients with PAD (ABI of $\leq$0.95), and once again found no difference in cardiovascular end points or improvement in intermittent claudication.[32]

Clopidogrel

Clopidogrel is a prodrug, metabolized by the liver, that irreversibly binds and inactivates the platelet receptor, $P2Y_{12}$. The Clopidogrel versus Aspirin in Patients at Risk of Ischaemic Events (CAPRIE) trial (n = 19,185) randomized patients with symptomatic atherosclerotic disease to clopidogrel 75 mg/d versus aspirin 325 mg/d. In the PAD subgroup (n = 6452), clopidogrel decreased MACE (relative risk reduction 23.8%; 95% CI, 8.9–36.2; P = .0028) compared with aspirin with similar bleeding rates.[33]

Ticagrelor

The EUCLID trial sought to build on the results of CAPRIE. Ticagrelor is also an inhibitor of the $P2Y_{12}$ platelet receptor but, unlike clopidogrel, is not a prodrug and does not require activation by the body. In this study, 13,885 patients with symptomatic PAD (ABI of <0.80 or prior revascularization) were randomized to either ticagrelor 90 mg or clopidogrel 75 mg/d. The primary end point of MACE was similar between groups (HR, 1.02; 95% CI, 0.92–1.13; P = .65) with no differences observed in the rates of acute limb ischemia (ALI) or lower limb revascularization.[34]

Vorapaxar

Vorapaxar is a novel antiplatelet drug that inhibits platelet aggregation by the irreversible inhibition of protease-activated receptor-1. In TRA 2°P-TIMI 50, 20,170 patients with stable atherosclerotic vascular disease (myocardial infarction, stroke, or symptomatic PAD) were randomized to vorapaxar 2.5 mg/d or placebo. Among the subgroup with PAD (n = 3787), there was no significant reduction in MACE with vorapaxar therapy (HR, 0.94; 95% CI, 0.78–1.14; P = .53), although there was a decrease in hospitalization for ALI (HR, 0.58; 95% CI, 0.39–0.86; P = .006) and peripheral artery revascularization (HR, 0.84; 95% CI, 0.73–0.97; P = .017). This came at the cost of increased bleeding with vorapaxar (HR, 1.62; 95% CI, 1.21–2.18; P = .001), which has in part limited the use of this drug.[35]

Dual antiplatelet therapy

The Clopidogrel for High Atherothrombotic Risk and Ischemic Stabilization, Management, and Avoidance trial (n = 15,603) evaluated the effect of low-dose aspirin plus clopidogrel versus aspirin plus placebo in individuals with stable cardiovascular disease or multiple risk factors. In subgroup analyses (n = 3096) of patients with symptomatic (92%) and asymptomatic (8%) PAD, there was similarly no decrease in MACE with dual antiplatelet therapy (DAPT) compared with aspirin (HR, 0.85; 95% CI, 0.66–1.08; P = .18).[36] Similar results were seen in the Clopidogrel and Acetylsalicylic Acid in Bypass Surgery trial in PAD patients undergoing unilateral surgical bypass grafting. Although there was no benefit to DAPT in decreasing mortality, the trial did suggest a benefit in decreasing prosthetic graft occlusions.[37]

Antithrombotic Therapy

Vitamin K antagonism

Until recently, data on antithrombotic therapy in PAD were largely limited to the Warfarin Antiplatelet Vascular Evaluation trial. In this study, 2161 patients with PAD were randomized to warfarin (international normalized ratio of 2–3) plus aspirin versus aspirin alone.[38] There was no significant reduction in MACE (relative risk, 0.92; 95% CI, 0.73–1.16; P = .48) with warfarin, although there was a significant increase in life-threatening bleeding (relative risk, 3.41; 95% CI, 1.84–6.35; P<.001). Accordingly, professional guidelines do not support the use of warfarin in treating PAD.[10]

Factor Xa inhibition

After the development of numerous oral factor Xa inhibitors, several trials has assessed their efficacy in reducing atherosclerotic events in conjunction with antiplatelet therapy. In the Cardiovascular Outcomes for People Using Anticoagulation Strategies (COMPASS) trial, 27,396 patients with stable CAD, PAD, or carotid disease were randomized to 1 of 3 drug regimens: the factor Xa inhibitor rivaroxaban 5 mg twice daily plus placebo, rivaroxaban 2.5 mg

Table 2
Antiplatelet and antithrombotic trials in patients with PAD

		Antiplatelet therapy				
Trial	POPADAD[31]	Aspirin for Asymptomatic Atherosclerosis Trialists[32]	CAPRIE[33]	CHARISMA[36]	EUCLID[34]	TRA 2°P-TIMI 50[35]
Intervention	Aspirin 100 mg/d vs placebo	Aspirin 100 mg/d vs placebo	Aspirin 325 mg/d vs clopidogrel 75 mg/d	Clopidogrel 75 mg/d plus either aspirin 75–162 mg/d or placebo	Ticagrelor 90 mg twice daily vs clopidogrel 75 mg/d	Vorapaxar 2.5 mg/d vs placebo
Study population	1276 patients with diabetes and an ABI of ≤ 0.99	3350 patients with an ABI of ≤0.95	19,185 total 6452 patients with intermittent claudication and either an ABI of ≤0.85 or prior revascularization/amputation	15,603 total 3096 patients with intermittent claudication and either an ABI of ≤0.85 or prior revascularization/amputation	13,885 patients with and ABI of ≤0.85 or prior revascularization	26,449 total 3787 patients with an ABI of ≤0.85 or prior revascularization
MACE outcomes	Vascular death, MI, stroke: HR, 0.98; 95% CI, 0.76–1.26	Fatal or nonfatal MI, stroke, or revascularization: HR, 1.03; 95% CI, 0.84–1.27	Vascular death, MI, or ischemic stroke in PAD subgroup: HR, 0.76; 95% CI, 0.64–0.91	CV death, MI, or stroke: HR, 0.85; 95% CI, 0.66–1.08	CV death, MI, or stroke: HR, 1.02; 95% CI, 0.92–1.13	CV death, MI, stroke: HR, 0.94; 95% CI, 0.78–1.14
MALE outcomes	Major amputation: 2% vs 2%	None reported	None reported	None reported	Hospitalization for ALI: HR, 1.03; 95% CI, 0.79–1.33 Lower limb revascularization: HR, 0.95; 95% CI, 0.90–1.05	Hospitalization for ALI: HR, 0.58; 95% CI, 0.39–0.86 Lower limb revascularization: HR, 0.84; 95% CI, 0.73–0.97

(continued on next page)

Table 2
(continued)

Trial	Antithrombotic therapy		
	WAVE[38]	COMPASS[40]	VOYAGER PAD[42]
Intervention	Warfarin with an INR goal of 2.0–3.0 plus antiplatelet monotherapy vs antiplatelet monotherapy alone	Rivaroxaban 2.5 mg twice daily plus aspirin 100 mg/d, rivaroxaban 5 mg twice daily plus placebo, or aspirin 100 mg/d plus placebo	Rivaroxaban 2.5 mg twice daily plus aspirin 100 mg/d vs aspirin plus placebo
Study population	2161 patients with symptomatic PAD or carotid/subclavian stenosis	27,395 7470 patients with symptomatic PAD or carotid stenosis	6564 patients with PAD and recent lower extremity revascularization
MACE outcomes	CV death, MI, stroke: RR, 0.92; 95% CI, 0.73–1.16	CV death, MI or stroke: ASA + rivaroxaban vs ASA + placebo: HR, 0.72; 95% CI, 0.57–0.90; $P = .0047$	Primary outcome MACE + MALE: HR, 0.85; 95% CI, 0.76–0.96
MALE outcomes	Revascularization: 3.3% vs 3.7%; $P = .64$ Amputation: 0.7% vs 1.1%; $P = .37$	MALE: HR, 0.54; 95% CI, 0.35–0.82; $P = .0037$	ALI: HR, 0.67; 95% CI, 0.55–0.82

Abbreviations: ABI, ankle-brachial index; ALI, acute limb ischemia; CAPRIE, Clopidogrel versus Aspirin in Patients at Risk of Ischaemic Events; CHARISMA, Clopidogrel for High Atherothrombotic Risk and Ischemic Stabilization, Management, and Avoidance; COMPASS, Cardiovascular Outcomes for People Using Anticoagulation Strategies; CV, cardiovascular; INR, international normalized ratio; MALE, major adverse limb event; MI, myocardial infarction; POPADAD, Progression of Arterial Disease and Diabetes; RR, relative risk; VOYAGER PAD, Vascular Outcomes Study of ASA Along with Rivaroxaban in Endovascular or Surgical Limb Revascularization for PAD; WAVE, Warfarin Antiplatelet Vascular Evaluation.

twice daily plus aspirin, or aspirin monotherapy plus placebo. The trial was terminated early after a mean follow-up period of 23 months owing to the decrease in MACE in the rivaroxaban plus aspirin versus the aspirin monotherapy group (HR, 0.76; 95% CI, 0.66–0.86; P<.001).[39]

The PAD subanalysis of COMPASS (n = 7470) included 4129 with symptomatic lower extremity PAD, 1422 patients with CAD and an ABI of less than 0.90, and 1919 patients with CAD and carotid disease. The combination of rivaroxaban plus aspirin compared with aspirin monotherapy showed significantly decreased rates of MACE (HR, 0.72; 95% CI, 0.57–0.90; P = .0047) and major adverse limb event (HR, 0.54; 95% CI, 0.35–0.82; P = .0037).[40] Similarly, this regimen led to decreases in ALI (HR, 0.56; 95% CI, 0.32–0.99; P = .04), vascular amputations (HR, 0.40; 95% CI, 0.20–0.79; P = .007), and peripheral vascular interventions (HR, 0.76; 95% CI, 0.60–0.97; P = .03).[40,41] Major bleeding was more common with the combination of low-dose rivaroxaban and aspirin (3.1% vs 1.9%, P = .009), but there was no increased risk in intracranial hemorrhage.[40]

To further evaluate the role of factor Xa inhibition in patients with PAD, the Vascular Outcomes Study of ASA Along with Rivaroxaban in Endovascular or Surgical Limb Revascularization for PAD (VOYAGER PAD) trial randomized 6564 patients with PAD who had undergone recent revascularization to rivaroxaban 2.5 mg twice daily plus aspirin versus aspirin alone. The addition of rivaroxaban led to a decrease in the primary outcome of MACE, ALI, or major amputation (HR, 0.85; 95% CI, 0.76–0.96; P = .009). The benefit for rivaroxaban was similar for endovascular and surgical revascularization and for revascularization for CLTI and non-CLTI. Bleeding risk was modestly increased (5.94% vs 4.06%; HR, 1.42; 95% CI, 1.10–1.84; P = .007) with no differences in life-threatening and intracranial hemorrhage.[42]

Antiplatelet and Antithrombotic Recommendations

The use of antiplatelet and antithrombotic in patients with PAD is based on multiple considerations including additional comorbidities, such as diabetes, the presence of polyvascular atherosclerotic disease, prior arterial revascularization, indications for therapeutic anticoagulation (eg, atrial fibrillation or venous thromboembolism), and other conditions that may further increase one's bleeding risk. This is an evolving field that is, not fully addressed in current professional guidelines. Our typical approach is as follows.

- For PAD without polyvascular disease or other risk factors, such as diabetes or prior

revascularization, use single antiplatelet therapy. Data suggest clopidogrel is more effective than aspirin.[33] Ticagrelor is a reasonable alternative to clopidogrel, particularly in poor metabolizers of clopidogrel.[34]
- In patients with symptomatic PAD and polyvascular disease, use aspirin plus low-dose rivaroxaban 2.5 mg twice daily.[40]
- After revascularization, DAPT to decrease instent thrombosis remains common practice, although data within a PAD population are limited.[43] Recent trial data support the use of aspirin plus low-dose rivaroxaban 2.5 mg twice daily after revascularization.[42] Additional studies are needed to compare DAPT to aspirin plus low-dose rivaroxaban after lower extremity percutaneous revascularization.
- In patients with lower extremity PAD but no attributable symptoms and no history of symptomatic atherosclerosis in other arterial beds, defer antiplatelet therapy.

OTHER THERAPIES
Cilostazol

Cilostazol is a selective inhibitor of phosphodiesterase III with antiplatelet, antithrombotic, and vasodilating properties. A meta-analysis (n = 2702) examining patients with stable, moderate to severe claudication from 8 randomized controlled trials found an increase in maximum walking distance by 50% and pain-free walking distance by 67% with cilostazol therapy.[44] Another meta-analysis (n = 1258) then compared cilostazol with placebo resulting in an improved maximum walking distance (50.7% vs 24.3%, P = .001) and pain-free walking distance (67.8% vs 42.6%, P = .0001).[45] Cilostazol is contraindicated in patients with heart failure owing to concerns of increased ventricular arrhythmias. Side effects of gastrointestinal intolerance, dizziness, and headaches may limit its use.[46,47]

Pentoxifylline

Pentoxifylline is a theophylline derivative initially studied to improve claudication symptoms. A randomized controlled trial comparing cilostazol, pentoxifylline, and placebo in patients with moderate to severe claudication found no difference in walking distance between pentoxifylline and placebo.[48] Current guidelines do not recommend the use of pentoxifylline for intermittent claudication.[10]

Recommendations

Cilostazol remains the only drug that has demonstrated efficacy in improving claudication symptoms with benefits seen 4 weeks after initiation, and guidelines recommend its use to improve walking distance and claudication symptoms.[10,45,49]

FUTURE DIRECTIONS

Given the results of COMPASS and VOYAGER PAD, we will likely have additional data for other factor Xa inhibitors as well as novel antithrombotic agents in the near future. There is ongoing work on new therapies to improve walking distance and claudication metrics. A pilot study of daily cocoa supplementation, which contains flavanols that may promote vascular growth and function, demonstrated improved walking distance and increased calf muscle perfusion on biopsy.[50,51] Anti-inflammatory drugs are also being explored as modulators of the proinflammatory pathways involved in the development and progression of atherosclerosis.[52] A small study exploring the effect of canakinumab, an interleukin 1β antagonist, in patients with PAD demonstrated improved pain free walking distance as early as 3 months after treatment.[51] We hopefully will have more cardiovascular outcome trial data, including limb events, of anti-inflammatory therapies in the coming years.

SUMMARY

The medical management options for PAD has improved markedly over the last 2 decades. In addition to standard risk modification therapies, advances have been made in improving lipid therapy with the addition of ezetimibe and PCSK9 inhibitors. More recently, this complex patient population has finally established an antiplatelet and antithrombic regimen that improves both MACE and major adverse limb event outcomes. We hope that the recent attention to PAD and limb outcomes leads to the development of novel therapies for this high risk patient population. Regardless, undertreatment remains a critical issue for patients with PAD, and an emphasis on both patient and provider awareness remains paramount.

CLINICS CARE POINTS

- Smoking cessation remains paramount in PAD, and varenicline should be used as a first-line therapy to help patients attain and maintain cessation.
- Statin therapy in PAD remains underused despite a lower risk of mortality and limb-related events regardless of baseline LDL-C levels. High-intensity statins are recommend in individuals with PAD.

- Angiotensin-converting enzyme inhibitors or angiotensin receptor blockers are first-line antihypertensive therapies in patients with PAD.
- A regimen of low-dose rivaroxaban 2.5 mg twice daily plus aspirin has both mortality and limb-related benefits in stable patients with PAD patients and following lower extremity revascularization.
- Cilostazol remains the only PAD therapy to improve walking distance and claudication symptoms.

DISCLOSURE

Dr Aday reports receiving consulting fees from OptumCare. Dr J. A. Gutierrez discloses the following relationships: research support from the Veterans Health Administration Career Development Award; consulting from Janssen Pharmaceuticals and Amgen Inc.

REFERENCES

1. Criqui MH, Aboyans V. Epidemiology of peripheral artery disease. Circ Res 2015;116(9):1509–26.
2. Gutierrez JA, Aday AW, Patel MR, et al. Polyvascular disease: reappraisal of the current clinical landscape. Circ Cardiovasc Interv 2019;12(12):e007385.
3. Willigendael EM, Teijink JA, Bartelink ML, et al. Influence of smoking on incidence and prevalence of peripheral arterial disease. J Vasc Surg 2004;40(6):1158–65.
4. Willigendael EM, Teijink JA, Bartelink ML, et al. Smoking and the patency of lower extremity bypass grafts: a meta-analysis. J Vasc Surg 2005;42(1):67–74.
5. Armstrong EJ, Wu J, Singh GD, et al. Smoking cessation is associated with decreased mortality and improved amputation-free survival among patients with symptomatic peripheral artery disease. J Vasc Surg 2014;60(6):1565–71.
6. Faulkner KW, House AK, Castleden WM. The effect of cessation of smoking on the accumulative survival rates of patients with symptomatic peripheral vascular disease. Med J Aust 1983;1(5):217–9.
7. Hennrikus D, Joseph AM, Lando HA, et al. Effectiveness of a smoking cessation program for peripheral artery disease patients: a randomized controlled trial. J Am Coll Cardiol 2010;56(25):2105–12.
8. Jorenby DE, Leischow SJ, Nides MA, et al. A controlled trial of sustained-release bupropion, a nicotine patch, or both for smoking cessation. N Engl J Med 1999;340(9):685–91.
9. Anthenelli RM, Benowitz NL, West R, et al. Neuropsychiatric safety and efficacy of varenicline, bupropion, and nicotine patch in smokers with and without psychiatric disorders (EAGLES): a double-blind,

randomised, placebo-controlled clinical trial. Lancet 2016;387(10037):2507–20.

10. Gerhard-Herman MD, Gornik HL, Barrett C, et al. 2016 AHA/ACC guideline on the management of patients with lower extremity peripheral artery disease: executive summary: a report of the American College of Cardiology/American Heart Association Task Force on Clinical Practice Guidelines. Circulation 2017;135(12):e686–725.

11. Barua RS, Rigotti NA, Benowitz NL, et al. 2018 ACC expert consensus decision pathway on tobacco cessation treatment: a report of the American College of Cardiology Task Force on Clinical Expert Consensus Documents. J Am Coll Cardiol 2018; 72(25):3332–65.

12. Aday AW, Everett BM. Dyslipidemia profiles in patients with peripheral artery disease. Curr Cardiol Rep 2019;21(6):42.

13. Heart Protection Study Collaborative G. Randomized trial of the effects of cholesterol-lowering with simvastatin on peripheral vascular and other major vascular outcomes in 20,536 people with peripheral arterial disease and other high-risk conditions. J Vasc Surg 2007;45(4):645–54. discussion 653-644.

14. Kumbhani DJ, Steg PG, Cannon CP, et al. Statin therapy and long-term adverse limb outcomes in patients with peripheral artery disease: insights from the REACH registry. Eur Heart J 2014;35(41): 2864–72.

15. Arya S, Khakharia A, Binney ZO, et al. Association of statin dose with amputation and survival in patients with peripheral artery disease. Circulation 2018; 137(14):1435–46.

16. Cannon CP, Blazing MA, Giugliano RP, et al. Ezetimibe added to statin therapy after acute coronary syndromes. N Engl J Med 2015;372(25):2387–97.

17. Bonaca MP, Nault P, Giugliano RP, et al. Low-density lipoprotein cholesterol lowering with evolocumab and outcomes in patients with peripheral artery disease: insights from the FOURIER trial (further cardiovascular outcomes research with PCSK9 inhibition in Subjects with elevated risk). Circulation 2018; 137(4):338–50.

18. Schwartz GG, Steg PG, Szarek M, et al. Peripheral artery disease and venous thromboembolic events after acute coronary syndrome. Circulation 2020; 141(20):1608–17.

19. Grundy SM, Stone NJ, Bailey AL, et al. 2018 AHA/ACC/AACVPR/AAPA/ABC/ACPM/ADA/AGS/APhA/ASPC/NLA/PCNA guideline on the management of blood cholesterol: a report of the American College of Cardiology/American Heart Association Task Force on Clinical Practice Guidelines. J Am Coll Cardiol 2019;73(24):e285–350.

20. Aboyans V, Ricco JB, Bartelink MEL, et al. 2017 ESC guidelines on the diagnosis and treatment of peripheral arterial diseases, in collaboration with the European Society for Vascular Surgery (ESVS): document covering atherosclerotic disease of extracranial carotid and vertebral, mesenteric, renal, upper and lower extremity arteries endorsed by: the European Stroke Organization (ESO)The Task Force for the Diagnosis and Treatment of Peripheral Arterial Diseases of the European Society of Cardiology (ESC) and of the European Society for Vascular Surgery (ESVS). Eur Heart J 2018;39(9):763–816.

21. Lewington S, Clarke R, Qizilbash N, et al. Age-specific relevance of usual blood pressure to vascular mortality: a meta-analysis of individual data for one million adults in 61 prospective studies. Lancet 2002;360(9349):1903–13.

22. Whelton PK, Carey RM, Aronow WS, et al. 2017 ACC/AHA/AAPA/ABC/ACPM/AGS/APhA/ASH/ASPC/NMA/PCNA guideline for the prevention, detection, evaluation, and management of high blood pressure in adults: a report of the American College of Cardiology/American Heart Association Task Force on Clinical Practice Guidelines. J Am Coll Cardiol 2018;71(19):e127–248.

23. Mehler PS, Coll JR, Estacio R, et al. Intensive blood pressure control reduces the risk of cardiovascular events in patients with peripheral arterial disease and type 2 diabetes. Circulation 2003;107(5):753–6.

24. Ostergren J, Sleight P, Dagenais G, et al. Impact of ramipril in patients with evidence of clinical or subclinical peripheral arterial disease. Eur Heart J 2004;25(1):17–24.

25. Fox KM, Investigators EUtOrocewPiscAd. Efficacy of perindopril in reduction of cardiovascular events among patients with stable coronary artery disease: randomised, double-blind, placebo-controlled, multicentre trial (the EUROPA study). Lancet 2003; 362(9386):782–8.

26. Investigators O, Yusuf S, Teo KK, et al. Telmisartan, ramipril, or both in patients at high risk for vascular events. N Engl J Med 2008;358(15):1547–59.

27. Bavry AA, Anderson RD, Gong Y, et al. Outcomes Among hypertensive patients with concomitant peripheral and coronary artery disease: findings from the INternational VErapamil-SR/Trandolapril STudy. Hypertension 2010;55(1):48–53.

28. Officers A, Coordinators for the ACRGTA, Lipid-Lowering Treatment to Prevent Heart Attack T. Major outcomes in high-risk hypertensive patients randomized to angiotensin-converting enzyme inhibitor or calcium channel blocker vs diuretic: the Antihypertensive and Lipid-Lowering Treatment to Prevent Heart Attack Trial (ALLHAT). JAMA 2002;288(23): 2981–97.

29. Fudim M, Hopley CW, Huang Z, et al. Association of hypertension and arterial blood pressure on limb and cardiovascular outcomes in symptomatic peripheral artery disease: the EUCLID trial. Circ Cardiovasc Qual Outcomes 2020;13(9):e006512.

30. Antithrombotic Trialists C. Collaborative meta-analysis of randomised trials of antiplatelet therapy for prevention of death, myocardial infarction, and stroke in high risk patients. BMJ 2002;324(7329):71–86.

31. Belch J, MacCuish A, Campbell I, et al. The prevention of progression of arterial disease and diabetes (POPADAD) trial: factorial randomised placebo controlled trial of aspirin and antioxidants in patients with diabetes and asymptomatic peripheral arterial disease. BMJ 2008;337:a1840.

32. Fowkes FG, Price JF, Stewart MC, et al. Aspirin for prevention of cardiovascular events in a general population screened for a low ankle brachial index: a randomized controlled trial. JAMA 2010;303(9):841–8.

33. Committee CS. A randomised, blinded, trial of clopidogrel versus aspirin in patients at risk of ischaemic events (CAPRIE). CAPRIE Steering Committee. Lancet 1996;348(9038):1329–39.

34. Hiatt WR, Fowkes FG, Heizer G, et al. Ticagrelor versus clopidogrel in symptomatic peripheral artery disease. N Engl J Med 2017;376(1):32–40.

35. Bonaca MP, Scirica BM, Creager MA, et al. Vorapaxar in patients with peripheral artery disease: results from TRA2{degrees}P-TIMI 50. Circulation 2013;127(14):1522–9, 1529.e1521-1526.

36. Cacoub PP, Bhatt DL, Steg PG, et al. Patients with peripheral arterial disease in the CHARISMA trial. Eur Heart J 2009;30(2):192–201.

37. Belch JJ, Dormandy J, Committee CW, et al. Results of the randomized, placebo-controlled clopidogrel and acetylsalicylic acid in bypass surgery for peripheral arterial disease (CASPAR) trial. J Vasc Surg 2010;52(4):825–33, 833.e821-822.

38. Warfarin Antiplatelet Vascular Evaluation Trial I, Anand S, Yusuf S, et al. Oral anticoagulant and antiplatelet therapy and peripheral arterial disease. N Engl J Med 2007;357(3):217–27.

39. Eikelboom JW, Connolly SJ, Bosch J, et al. Rivaroxaban with or without aspirin in stable cardiovascular disease. N Engl J Med 2017;377(14):1319–30.

40. Anand SS, Bosch J, Eikelboom JW, et al. Rivaroxaban with or without aspirin in patients with stable peripheral or carotid artery disease: an international, randomised, double-blind, placebo-controlled trial. Lancet 2018;391(10117):219–29.

41. Anand SS, Caron F, Eikelboom JW, et al. Major adverse limb events and mortality in patients with peripheral artery disease. J Am Coll Cardiol 2018; 71(20):2306–15.

42. Bonaca MP, Bauersachs RM, Anand SS, et al. Rivaroxaban in peripheral artery disease after revascularization. N Engl J Med 2020;382(21):1994–2004.

43. Aday AW, Gutierrez JA. Antiplatelet therapy following peripheral arterial interventions: the choice is yours. Circ Cardiovasc Interv 2020;13(8):e009727.

44. Thompson PD, Zimet R, Forbes WP, et al. Meta-analysis of results from eight randomized, placebo-controlled trials on the effect of cilostazol on patients with intermittent claudication. Am J Cardiol 2002; 90(12):1314–9.

45. Pande RL, Hiatt WR, Zhang P, et al. A pooled analysis of the durability and predictors of treatment response of cilostazol in patients with intermittent claudication. Vasc Med 2010;15(3):181–8.

46. Regensteiner JG, Ware JE Jr, McCarthy WJ, et al. Effect of cilostazol on treadmill walking, community-based walking ability, and health-related quality of life in patients with intermittent claudication due to peripheral arterial disease: meta-analysis of six randomized controlled trials. J Am Geriatr Soc 2002; 50(12):1939–46.

47. Lee C, Nelson PR. Effect of cilostazol prescribed in a pragmatic treatment program for intermittent claudication. Vasc Endovascular Surg 2014;48(3): 224–9.

48. Dawson DL, Cutler BS, Hiatt WR, et al. A comparison of cilostazol and pentoxifylline for treating intermittent claudication. Am J Med 2000;109(7):523–30.

49. Beebe HG, Dawson DL, Cutler BS, et al. A new pharmacological treatment for intermittent claudication: results of a randomized, multicenter trial. Arch Intern Med 1999;159(17):2041–50.

50. McDermott MM, Criqui MH, Domanchuk K, et al. Cocoa to improve walking performance in older people with peripheral artery disease: the COCOA-PAD pilot randomized clinical trial. Circ Res 2020;126(5): 589–99.

51. Russell KS, Yates DP, Kramer CM, et al. A randomized, placebo-controlled trial of canakinumab in patients with peripheral artery disease. Vasc Med 2019;24(5):414–21.

52. Camara Planek MI, Silver AJ, Volgman AS, et al. Exploratory review of the role of statins, colchicine, and aspirin for the prevention of radiation-associated cardiovascular disease and mortality. J Am Heart Assoc 2020;9(2):e014668.

53. Hartmann-Boyce J, Chepkin SC, Ye W, et al. Nicotine replacement therapy versus control for smoking cessation. Cochrane Database Syst Rev 2018;5: CD000146.

54. Bolliger CT, Zellweger JP, Danielsson T, et al. Smoking reduction with oral nicotine inhalers: double blind, randomised clinical trial of efficacy and safety. BMJ 2000;321(7257):329–33.

55. Croghan IT, Hurt RD, Dakhil SR, et al. Randomized comparison of a nicotine inhaler and bupropion for smoking cessation and relapse prevention. Mayo Clin Proc 2007;82(2):186–95.

56. Fiore MC, Smith SS, Jorenby DE, et al. The effectiveness of the nicotine patch for smoking cessation. A meta-analysis. JAMA 1994;271(24):1940–7.

57. Mohammadi D. Black-box warnings could be removed from varenicline. Lancet Respir Med 2016;4(11):861.

Revascularization Strategies for Acute and Chronic Limb Ischemia

Jocelyn M. Beach, MD, MS

KEYWORDS

- Acute limb ischemia • Chronic limb ischemia • CLI • CTLI • ALI • Endovascular • Surgical bypass
- Revascularization

KEY POINTS

- There are few high-quality data guiding the best interventional approach for the treatment of chronic limb-threatening ischemia.
- Decisions regarding endovascular or open interventions should be made based on evaluation of patient risk and functional status, lesion anatomy, extent of wound, and availability of conduit.
- Acute limb ischemia is a clinical diagnosis requiring a high index of suspicion. Any delay in identification and treatment can lead to increased risk of limb loss and mortality.
- Patients with limb ischemia frequently have concomitant comorbidities that require intensive medical therapies to decrease the risk of major adverse cardiac and limb events.

INTRODUCTION

Patients with limb ischemia, both in the acute (<2 weeks) and chronic (≥2 weeks) setting, are at significantly increased risk of limb loss, adverse cardiovascular events, and death. Chronic limb-threatening ischemia (CLTI) is present in 12% of the US population, and the costs are high, both socially and economically. Patients with CLTI have 1- and 5-year mortality rates of 20% and 50%, respectively.[1] Those with CLTI who go untreated have a 22% major amputation rate at 1 year.[2] Those with acute limb ischemia (ALI) have similar long-term risk of mortality, although a much higher 15% to 20% postoperative risk of death.[1] This review focuses on revascularization strategies in patients with CLTI and ALI, highlighting the need to treat the entire patient, addressing comorbidities, smoking cessation, and other risk factors, in addition to treatment of the ischemic limb.

Revascularization of a given patient's ischemic extremity is complex, with decisions requiring consideration of patient risk, severity of limb ischemia, and anatomic complexity. Both endovascular and open surgical approaches should be considered, with anatomic and patient factors guiding these decisions. Few studies comparing these approaches have been performed and more are ongoing, both in the acute[3–5] and chronic settings.[6–8] Factors that should be considered to guide these decisions are discussed in detail.

CHRONIC LIMB-THREATENING ISCHEMIA

New terminology, CLTI, was presented in the 2019 Global Vascular Guidelines to replace critical limb ischemia to better reflect the broader group of patients with advanced lower limb ischemia, wounds, neuropathy, and infection This includes patients with advanced peripheral artery disease (PAD) with rest pain, gangrene, or ulceration of greater than 2 weeks duration.[9] The goals of revascularization in patients with CTLI are to minimize tissue loss and decrease the risks of amputation and mortality[9,10] by treating hemodynamically significant stenosis. In patients with tissue loss, it is important to restore in-line and pulsatile flow

Section of Vascular Surgery, Heart and Vascular Institute, Dartmouth-Hitchcock Medical Center, 1 Medical Center Drive, Lebanon, NH 03756, USA
E-mail address: jocelyn.m.beach@hitchcock.org

Cardiol Clin 39 (2021) 483–494
https://doi.org/10.1016/j.ccl.2021.06.006
0733-8651/21/© 2021 Elsevier Inc. All rights reserved.

to the foot. Endovascular, open surgical, and hybrid approaches should be considered to achieve these goals. There has been increased recognition that management decisions for patients with CLTI should not be based on the lesion or degree of ischemia alone. The Society for Vascular Surgery Threatened Limb Classification system is a validated tool based on extent of wound, ischemia, and foot infection (WIfI) to help risk stratify and guide revascularization strategies in these complex patients (**Fig. 1**).[11] The WIfI system correlates with risk of major amputation and wound healing, as well as the effectiveness of revascularization strategies.[11–13]

There is a lack of high-quality evidence directly comparing revascularization strategies for CLTI. Currently enrolling trials such as Best Endovascular versus Best Surgical Therapy for Patients with Critical Limb Ischemia (BEST-CLI),[6,8] Bypass versus Angioplasty in Severe Ischaemia of the Leg (BASIL-2),[14] and Balloon versus Stenting in Severe Ischaemia of the Leg (BASIL-3) trials will provide important evidence to guide management of this challenging population, particularly with regard to infrainguinal disease. With the current paucity of high-quality data, the choice of treatment strategy should weigh each approach's durability, invasiveness, and technical feasibility in context of patient risk factors, anatomy, and limb classification criteria described elsewhere in this article.

Patient Evaluation

A thorough patient evaluation is the first step to guiding therapy for CLTI. A detailed history should focus on cardiovascular risk factors, prior therapies and vascular interventions, details regarding the timing and evolution of symptoms, and assessment of wounds and infection. Assessment of functional and ambulatory status is critical. After a complete evaluation, the physician should estimate a patient's periprocedural risk and life expectancy.[15,16] The revascularization strategy for the same wound in an ambulatory patient with low perioperative risk may be different from a bedridden patient in whom estimated 2-year survival is 50% or less.

All patients with concern for CLTI should have ankle pressures and ankle–brachial index measurements performed. In those with CLTI and tissue loss, the addition of toe pressure measurements and toe–brachial indices can be valuable.[9,17] Noninvasive imaging is recommended before catheter-based angiography. In patients with diminished or nonpalpable femoral pulses, computed tomography arteriography (CTA) is preferred to assess for evidence of aortoiliac or inflow disease. Infrainguinal disease can be assessed with duplex ultrasound examination, CTA, or magnetic resonance angiography. Noninvasive imaging can be often used to select treatment strategy with diagnostic angiography

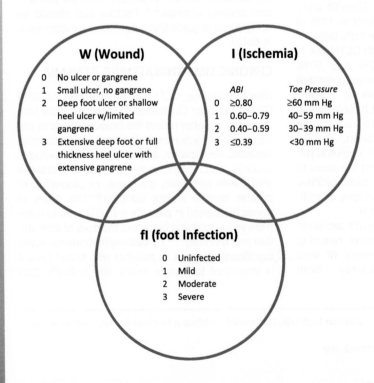

Fig. 1. Society for Vascular Surgery Lower Extremity Limb (SVS WIfI) classification system.[11] ABI, ankle–brachial index. (*Data from* Boulton AJM, Armstrong DG, Kirsner RS, Attinger CE, Lavery LA, Lipsky BA, Mills JL, Steinberg JS. Diagnosis and Management of Diabetic Foot Complications. American Diabetes Association, Arlington (VA), 2018.)

W (Wound)

0 No ulcer or gangrene
1 Small ulcer, no gangrene
2 Deep foot ulcer or shallow heel ulcer w/limited gangrene
3 Extensive deep foot or full thickness heel ulcer with extensive gangrene

I (Ischemia)

	ABI	Toe Pressure
0	≥0.80	≥60 mm Hg
1	0.60–0.79	40–59 mm Hg
2	0.40–0.59	30–39 mm Hg
3	≤0.39	<30 mm Hg

fI (foot Infection)

0 Uninfected
1 Mild
2 Moderate
3 Severe

performed as part of a planned therapeutic endovascular intervention. In some situations, diagnostic angiography can be helpful to select a distal target in preparation for open bypass. Vein mapping should be performed for all patients who are candidates for surgical bypass.[18]

Level of Disease

Identification of levels of disease is necessary to formulate a revascularization strategy. Patients with CLTI often have multilevel disease, and often will require treatment of both inflow (aortoiliac and femoral), and outflow (femoropopliteal and tibioperoneal disease). This point is particularly true of patients with wounds, in whom it is important to achieve in-line pulsatile flow to the foot. Inflow should always be addressed first in patients with rest pain; this intervention may be the only one required if severe disease is present and treated successfully. At all anatomic levels of disease, there are both open and endovascular, as well as hybrid approaches, to achieve in-line flow, as discussed elsewhere in this article.

Endovascular Revascularization

The development of endovascular therapies for PAD have significantly impacted the treatment of aortoiliac occlusive disease. As compared with invasive aortobifemoral bypass, even long segment Trans Atlantic Society Consensus (TASC) C and even D occlusive iliac lesions can be successfully treated with angioplasty and stenting percutaneously or with or without addition of femoral endarterectomies (**Fig. 2**). Assessment with CTA is invaluable for planning. Aortic bifurcation lesions are traditionally treated with 'kissing' balloon expandable stents to protect the contralateral iliac. Balloon expandable stents are selected for precise delivery and high hoop strength to treat calcific disease, with some operators favoring stent grafts for TASC C and D lesions.[19] External iliac disease is also best treated with stenting, though self-expanding stents are often adequate. This disease process often extends into the common femoral vessels and can effectively be treated with concomitant endarterectomy. Patency rates are excellent for TASC A and B lesions with primary assisted patency rate of 71% at 10 years, and is comparable with open surgical revascularization. For TASC C and D lesions, primary and secondary patency at 5 years is 60% to 86% and 80% to 98%, respectively.[20]

Occlusive disease of the superficial femoral artery and popliteal artery can be approached with endovascular therapies. TASC[1] and now Global Limb Anatomic Staging System[9] anatomic staging can help to distinguish which lesions may be treated successfully with an endovascular approach. Balloon angioplasty alone has a high initial success rates, particularly for short lesions, however 1-year primary patency rates are low at 47% to 63%. For lesions greater than 10 cm, flow-limiting dissections, or residual stenosis after angioplasty, stenting improves 3-year primary patency to approximately 65%.[21] Drug-coated angioplasty balloons (DCB) have been primarily studied in patients with claudication, and there are few data in patients with patients with CLTI. DCBs are associated with increased patency and total lesion revascularization when compared with angioplasty alone.[22–24] Drug-coated stents are also primarily studied in patients with claudication; the 5-year patency is significantly higher for DCBs as compared with angioplasty for TASC C/D lesions, at 66.4% versus

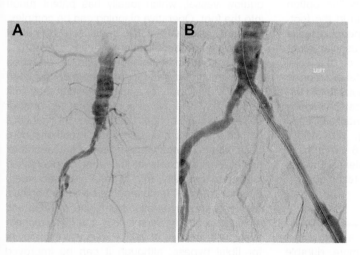

Fig. 2. Hybrid revascularization of occlusive iliofemoral disease. (*A*) Digital subtraction angiography (DSA) noting chronic occlusion of left common iliac with near occlusion of external iliac through length. (*B*) DSA after the patient underwent left common iliac and external iliac artery stenting with femoral endarterectomy and bovine patch angioplasty.

43.4%, respectively.[25] There has been significant controversy regarding an increased mortality signal identified in meta-analysis of randomized controlled trials (RCTs) investigating paclitaxel-coated balloons and stents.[26] Several analyses based on patient-level data have not confirmed these findings and do not prove increased mortality with DCB or drug-eluting stents.[27–29]

Endovascular treatment of tibial vessels primarily uses angioplasty with good results. These vessels are most often treated with small 2- to 3-mm angioplasty balloons in long lengths to address often diffuse disease. The efficacy of DCBs has been compared with conventional angioplasty in limited RCTs. Compared with conventional angioplasty, accelerated wound healing was noted with DCBs in the ACHILLES trial,[30,31] but not in the IN.PACT DEEP trial, in which there was a trend toward increased major amputation with DCBs[32]

Adjunctive debulking devices such as excisional and rotational atherectomy devices can be helpful, particularly in heavily calcified lesions. Several RCTs have evaluated these devices. The DEFINITIVE LE trial showed a limb salvage rate of 95% and primary patency of 71% with atherectomy in patients with CLTI,[33] which was comparable with angioplasty and infrainguinal stenting. There is a risk that distal embolization from these devices can complicate treatment.

There is limited evidence regarding angiosome directed therapy, which suggests that patency of the pedal loop may improve wound healing. Advocates suggest that wound healing can improve with the establishment of direct flow into the infrapopliteal vessel most directly perfusing the location of wound on the foot.[34,35] A recent meta-analysis of several small studies noted improved wound healing and limb salvage, but acknowledged the available evidence is of poor quality.[36]

Some patients are referred to as "no option CLTI" without any identifiable vessel in the foot, typically with extensive tibial and pedal disease not amenable to traditional endovascular techniques or bypass owing to the absence of a distal target. Percutaneous deep vein arterialization is performed by creating an arteriovenous fistula using stent grafts to retrograde perfuse the venous system in the foot after lysing the venous valves.[37] Preliminary data are encouraging, with 100% amputation free survival at 6 months.[38] PROMISE-II is prospective multicenter pivotal trial is currently enrolling evaluating this technique.

Open Surgical Revascularization

Surgical revascularization options at most anatomic levels of disease are more durable compared with endovascular approaches. This process is at the cost of increased periprocedural risk including myocardial infarction, bleeding, surgical site complications, and death. In patients with a low surgical risk and life expectancy of more than 2 years, the durability of an open intervention may be favored.

For the treatment of severe aortoiliac occlusive disease as described by TASC C and D lesions,[1] the gold standard of therapy is aortobifemoral bypass, which requires bilateral groin incisions and a laparotomy. The infrarenal aorta and bilateral iliac artery segments are replaced with a prosthetic graft, and are often combined with femoral or profunda endarterectomies to ensure patent outflow. This option is a durable one for appropriately selected patients, with 5- and 10-year patency rates of 95% and 85% to 90%, respectively.[39,40] Alternatively, higher risk patients who are not able to be treated with endovascular approaches can be treated with axillary–bifemoral artery bypass. Patency for this extra-anatomic reconstruction is significantly lower with 3-year patency rates of 50% to 85%; however, it avoids the perioperative risks associated with laparotomy and aortic clamping.

Femoral and profunda femoral disease is best treated with open endarterectomy with bovine or synthetic patch angioplasty for durable, long-term patency (>90%).[41] Open surgical repair is far preferred in this location to debulk what are typically heavily calcified lesions and to visualize the profunda femoral and superficial femoral artery origins to ensure their patency. These procedures are highly effective with a low risk of complications.

Open surgical repair of infrainguinal disease is performed with lower extremity bypass, providing direct inline flow through a conduit to a patent outflow vessel, which ideally has patent runoff into the foot. Operative planning can be complex, requiring adequate inflow, selection of patent outflow, and identification of an appropriate bypass conduit. Autologous vein is preferred over a prosthetic graft for improved patency; however, the availability of a suitable length may limit options.[42,43] The use of contralateral leg, arm, or spliced vein are options, particularly if distal tibial or pedal targets are necessary. Prosthetic conduits with polytetrafluoroethylene are acceptable; however, they come at the cost of decreased long-term durability, with 1- and 3-year secondary patency rates for femoral to below-knee popliteal bypass with polytetrafluoroethylene of 68% and 44%, respectively, versus 96% and 86%, respectively, with the use of vein. Patency is even lower for tibial bypass, although it can be improved with the use of vein cuffs. The overall improved long-term patency can come at an upfront cost of prolonged recovery and wound healing.[44]

Results of Open Surgical Versus Endovascular Interventions for Chronic Limb-Threatening Ischemia

There is significant debate regarding the best approach for the treatment of CLTI, and this is in part owing to the lack of high-quality data to address this complex but important question. The Bypass versus Angioplasty in Severe Ischaemia of the Leg (BASIL) trial[7,45] is one of the few RCTs comparing angioplasty alone with open surgical bypass in patients with severe CLTI and infrainguinal disease that could be treated with either approach. The early amputation-free survival was similar; however, those who survived more than 2 years and were randomized to surgery had significantly improved survival with a mean follow-up of 3.1 years (range, 1.0–5.7 years) and trended toward improved amputation-free survival.[46] Interestingly, mortality was worst in patients who required surgical bypass after failed angioplasty,[47] suggesting that an endovascular-first approach is not without cost.

We await data from aforementioned ongoing RCTs to help guide decisions. At present, both options, including hybrid approaches, should be considered in these complex decisions weighing patient risk, anatomy, wound, and availability of conduit. The absence of quality vein or a high-risk patient comorbidity profile encourage a more aggressive endovascular strategy, whereas a patient with long, complex lesions and excellent vein conduit may benefit from the longevity of an open bypass.

Amputation

Limb preservation is the primary objective in the treatment of most patients with CTLI. For some patients, however, amputation may ultimately be necessary despite revascularization; for other patients, it may be the most appropriate primary therapy. In those with a limited life expectancy, nonambulatory status, or an unsalvageable limb, primary major amputation or palliative care should be considered in shared decision-making with patient. In some patient cohorts, amputation may be associated with improved quality of life.[48]

ACUTE LIMB ISCHEMIA

ALI is a medical emergency and characterized by less than 2 weeks of symptoms, which can include pallor, pulselessness, poikilothermia, paresthesia, and paralysis of the affected extremity.[49,50] Early presentation with urgent evaluation and diagnosis are critical to avoid permanent neuromotor deficits and limb loss.[51] High limb loss mortality rates are driven primarily by delayed time to revascularization, and comorbid conditions. The 5-year mortality and amputation rates are high, at 54% and 28%, respectively.

Patient Evaluation

ALI is a clinical diagnosis. A history of arrhythmias, recent myocardial infarction, infection, malignancy, hypercoagulable states, and PAD or vascular interventions should be discussed. A thorough vascular examination evaluating pulses and Doppler signals from arteries in the affected and contralateral limbs should be performed and can help to identify the level of disease. A motor and sensory examination of the leg, especially of the foot and digits, will identify cases of more severe ischemia and define the urgency of revascularization.

The etiology of ALI is most often thrombotic; however, embolic causes also should be considered, especially in the absence of PAD and when contralateral distal pulses are palpable. Findings from the history and examination can often suggest the cause of ALI, but definitively determining the etiology should not delay treatment. After urgent revascularization, the evaluation should include an electrocardiogram to evaluate for arrhythmia, echocardiogram to evaluate for valvular disease or left ventricular thrombus, and CTA of the aorta to evaluate for aortic thrombus.[10,52]

Treatment Selection

Patients with ALI are categorized by their clinical signs and symptoms as described by Rutherford (**Table 1**).[53] Class I patients have a limb that is not immediately threatened. These patients can often be treated with systemic anticoagulation alone, at least initially. Some require interval intervention with either open or endovascular approaches, based on the patient's comorbidities, etiology of ischemia, and the presence of prior underlying PAD.

Those with Class II ischemia have the greatest opportunity for improvement and limb salvage if ALI recognized and treated in a timely fashion. Class IIA ischemia is a marginally threatened limb that requires urgent intervention and is characterized by mild sensory changes in the digits without any motor deficits. Endovascular or open approaches can be considered; however, percutaneous therapies are more successful when

Table 1
Clinical categories of ALI

Category	Description	Findings		Doppler Examination	
		Sensory Loss	Motor Loss	Arterial	Venous
I: Viable	Not immediately threatened	None	None	Audible	Audible
II: Threatened					
IIA: Marginally	Salvageable if promptly treated	Minimal (toes) or none	None	Inaudible	Audible
IIB: Immediately	Salvageable with immediate revascularization	More than toes with rest pain	Mild, moderate	Inaudible	Audible
III: Irreversible	Major tissue loss or permanent nerve damage inevitable	Profound, anesthetic	Profound, paralysis (rigor)	Inaudible	Inaudible

From Rutherford RB, Baker JD, Ernst C, et al. Recommended standards for reports dealing with lower extremity ischemia: revised version. *J Vasc Surg*. 1997;26(3):517-538.

performed less than 14 days after symptom onset. These limbs do not require immediate restoration of flow and can typically tolerate thrombolytic infusion that occurs over hours. In contrast, Class IIB ischemia involves an immediately threatened limb with motor deficits and/or more severe sensory symptoms. Without emergent revascularization, these patients have a high risk of limb loss. In general, open surgical approaches are performed to emergently restore arterial flow.

Those with Class III ischemia have irreversible ischemia with severe motor and sensory deficits, often owing to delayed presentation or diagnosis. There is no benefit to revascularization in these patients and these limbs should be treated with primary amputation to prevent systemic metabolic complications.

Endovascular Approaches

Percutaneous endovascular approaches provide a minimally invasive method to address patients with ALI. Catheter-directed thrombolysis (CDT) is the most commonly used technique; however, the evolution of devices with mechanical and suction thrombectomy capabilities have expanded endovascular therapies for ALI to enable more rapid restoration of flow. The objective of these therapies is to remove the acute occlusive thromboembolic disease, and in the setting of acute thrombosis, uncover the inciting lesion. This lesion can then be address by standard endovascular techniques for treatment of PAD.

Catheter-directed thrombolysis
Catheter-directed intra-arterial infusion of thrombolytic agents has become an invaluable tool in the treatment of ALI. For many practitioners, this technique is the preferred therapy for the treatment of patients with Class I and IIA ALI who can tolerate a slow restoration of perfusion. From a percutaneous approach, diagnostic imaging is obtained of the affected limb to identify the occlusive lesion of concern. This lesion is then crossed with a wire and, after confirmation of access in the true lumen distally, an infusion catheter is placed. These catheters have multiple side holes and a valve at the end to ensure infusion of thrombolytic agent through the side holes. The catheter length is selected to span across the occlusion from patent vessel proximally to distally. A thrombolytic agent, such as tissue plasminogen activator, is then infused at a rate of 0.5 to 1.0 mg/h through the catheter for 6 to 24 hours with 300 to 500 U/h of heparin infused through the sheath to prevent thrombosis. Repeat angiography is planned within 6 to 24 hours to assess progress. If repeat angiography suggests that the patient may benefit from additional lysis and there are no complications, the infusion can continue with the plan for a second repeat lysis check. Residual lesions can be addressed with standard endovascular techniques.

Before the initiation of lysis, patients should be screened for contraindications to thrombolysis, which place them at high risk of bleeding events. During the infusion, patients are monitored closely in an intensive care setting with trending of blood counts and coagulation factors, including fibrinogen. A decrease in fibrinogen may indicate increased systemic fibrinolysis and should trigger return for angiography and possible cessation or decrease in the rate of lytic infusion.

Several prospective, randomized clinical trials have evaluated the usefulness of CDT compared with open revascularization for ALI, and found similar limb salvage rates.[3–5] CDT is effective at clearing thrombus in 75% to 92% patients. The University of Rochester trial noted a higher 1-year mortality rate in the surgical arm compared with CDT (58% vs 84%) owing to in-hospital cardiopulmonary complications.[5] The STILE trial noted lower amputation rates in patients treated with CDT compared with surgery if treated within 14 days of symptoms (11% vs 30%), but higher (12% vs 3%) after 14 days.[3] In the TOPAS trial, patients presenting within 14 days of symptoms had similar in-hospital and 6-month amputation rates between CDT and surgery (72% vs 75%).[4] A meta-analysis of 10 studies evaluating CDT showed a high technical success rate of approximately 80%, but also a 29% risk of perioperative complications, and approximately 12% risk of amputation and approximately 4% risk of 30-day mortality.[54]

Percutaneous pharmacomechanical and mechanical thrombectomy

There are several devices aimed at mechanically disrupting thrombus to attempt to accelerate speed of thrombolysis. The AngioJet Thrombectomy System (Medrad International, Indianola, PA) is most commonly used device in this setting with the ability to act as a pharmacomechanical device with its power pulse mode. Using this feature, tissue plasminogen activator (tPA) is sprayed through the catheter into the thrombus and allowed to dwell. The liquefied thrombus is removed by high-velocity saline jet that creates a Venturi effect at the catheter tip, resulting in fragmentation and aspiration of thrombus.

The Trellis Peripheral Infusion System (Bacchus Vascular Inc, Santa Clara, CA) consists of an over-the-wire device with 2 compliant balloons that, when inflated, aim to isolate the zone of treatment. The thrombolytic drugs can be infused into this segment and an oscillation wire can be activated to mechanically disrupt and liquefy thrombus. This thrombus is then able to be aspirated through the sheath after deflation of the distal balloon.

The EKOS EndoWave Infusion Catheter (Boston Scientific, Marlborough, MA) uses ultrasound to increase penetration of thrombolytic agents into the thrombus. Several RCTs have compared this technique with standard CDT, noting a decreased thrombolysis time tPA and dose reduction with no difference in bleeding events.[55]

The thrombus can also be removed using aspiration mechanical thrombectomy devices. These specialty catheters are advanced over the wire and thrombus aspiration is performed using various techniques, including manual and hand-held aspiration as well as continuous vacuum as used with the Indigo (Penumbra Inc, Alameda, CA) device. These catheters have moderate effectiveness[56] and are most effective in treating small and distal thrombus, because they are limited by the size of the catheter.

The benefit of these devices is the rapid removal of thrombus and the ability to restore perfusion in a single setting. If successful, these devices can decrease the need for open surgical intervention in some patients with Class IIB ischemia who would not tolerate CDT alone or in patients with contraindications to lysis. These devices can also help to create a flow channel and decrease thrombus burden and ischemia, acting as an adjunct to CDT to resolve any residual thrombus with favorable short- and long-term results.[57,58]

Open Surgical Approaches

The rapid restoration of perfusion can be achieved with open surgical intervention. This goal can be of critical importance in patients with Class IIB ischemia, who cannot tolerate the additional ischemia time required during the infusion of lytic agents or if alternative endovascular therapies are unsuccessful in restoring adequate perfusion. These surgical techniques overlap with those used in CTLI, with the addition of catheter thrombectomy or embolectomy to remove acute occlusive emboli or thrombus. After the removal of the acute occlusive disease, the inciting lesion is then treated with endarterectomy, surgical bypass, or using a hybrid approach.

Balloon catheter thromboembolectomy

The mainstay of open therapy for ALI is balloon catheter thromboembolectomy, first described in 1963 by Fogarty and colleagues.[59] After exposure and control of the vessel of interest, a catheter with an inflatable balloon at the end is passed antegrade and retrograde through an arteriotomy or graftotomy with the balloon deflated. Once the catheter is past the occlusive lesion, the balloon is inflated and carefully withdrawn, extracting any thrombus or clot within the vessel through the arteriotomy. Successful thromboembolectomy clears the embolism or thrombus, with a return of forward and back bleeding from the vessel. Direct intra-arterial infusion of thrombolytics can supplement this procedure, particularly to address small vessels and distal thrombosis. If treating an acute embolic event, this procedure may be the only necessary intervention. With a thrombotic event, angiography should be performed to identify and plan to treat the inciting lesion.

Surgical bypass and endarterectomy

Shorter lesions limited to a single vessel can be treated with an endarterectomy with patch angioplasty. Most commonly, this technique is used to treat the femoral artery in the setting of in-site thrombosis of a preexisting stenosis (**Fig. 3**). In patients with a failed attempt at balloon thrombectomy or in those with long-segment occlusive lesions and preexisting PAD, an open surgical bypass can be performed with similar principles described previously to provide arterial flow from an open inflow source to a patent outflow vessel bypassing around an occlusive lesion. Popliteal artery aneurysms can cause ALI by embolization of thrombus within the aneurysm or by acute occlusion and embolization of the aneurysm. Popliteal artery aneurysms also can be treated with open bypass after restoration of outflow. In the treatment of these aneurysms, it is essential to ligate the popliteal artery proximal and distal to the aneurysm just proximal to the distal anastomosis to prevent further embolization. Otherwise, the technical principles are similar for these procedures as for CLTI.

Fasciotomy

Fasciotomies should be considered in all patients presenting with ALI to prevent and treat compartment syndrome. Following reperfusion after prolonged ischemia, swelling of the skeletal muscle and soft tissues occurs, increasing the pressure within the lower extremity compartments. Compartment pressures of greater than 30 mm Hg result in compression of the capillaries and venules, impeding venous outflow and leading to muscle malperfusion.

Patients at the highest risk for compartment syndrome are those with Class IIB ischemia, and those with reperfusion more than 4 to 6 hours after symptoms and rapid restoration of flow.[9,10,50] Patients with Class IIB ischemia should receive prophylactic 4-compartment fasciotomies after revascularization. All patients treated for ALI should be monitored serially after reperfusion for signs and symptoms of compartment syndrome. Clinicians should have a high index of suspicion and low threshold to perform fasciotomies in these patients because there is a narrow window before nerve injury and muscle death occurs.

Outcomes of Acute Limb Ischemia

Outcomes in patients presenting with ALI are humbling and have not improved significantly over time. Prolonged ischemia is associated with worse outcomes, both in-hospital and at 1 year. At 1 year, amputation rates range from 7% to 26%, with an increased risk of a higher level of amputation required as compared with patients with CTLI.[5,60,61] Mortality at 1 year is 10% to 22%, and in open subgroup from Ouriel and colleagues as high as 42%.[5,61,62] Patients with ALI have more significant comorbidities as compared with patients with CTLI, likely influencing this high rate.[60]

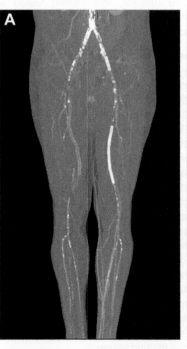 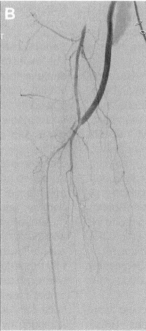

Fig. 3. Vascular imaging of a patient who presented with acute onset of right lower extremity rest pain with sensory and mild motor deficits (class IIB ischemia). (*A*) Preoperative CTA noting acute occlusion of right common femoral artery and femoral to above knee popliteal artery bypass with polytetrafluoroethylene. (*B*) Digital subtraction arteriogram after completion of right femoral endarterectomy and profundaplasty with redo femoral to now below knee popliteal artery bypass now showing runoff to anterior tibial artery.

At 2 years, up to 11% of patients will have recurrent ALI.[49]

POSTREVASCULARIZATION MANAGEMENT

Revascularization of limbs in patients treated for either acute limb-threatening ischemia or CLTI is critical to achieve limb salvage and improve survival. Still, these patients require aggressive secondary prevention therapies to decrease the risk of adverse cardiovascular and cerebrovascular events. Antiplatelet agents, high-intensity statins, smoking cessation, and continued management of underlying comorbidities are important.[9,10] In patients with CLTI, multidisciplinary care is imperative to achieve the best outcomes. For patients with concomitant wounds, appropriate wound care, infection control, and offloading are imperative. Independent of revascularization technique, long-tern surveillance should be performed to ensure long-term limb salvage and continue wound healing. Every follow-up should include a clinical and complete pulse examination. The ankle–brachial index and toe pressures should be monitored, and a decrease of more than 0.15 in ankle–brachial index or new symptoms or wound should trigger further evaluation. Duplex ultrasound surveillance should be performed on bypasses to evaluate for the development of stenosis to maintain long-term patency.[9] Even after successful revascularization, patients with CLTI continue to have a long-term risk for reintervention, failure of revascularization, and amputation and therefore require often life-long attention.

CLINICS CARE POINTS

- Patients with acute and chronic limb ischemia have high rate of limb loss and mortality with late mortality driven by preexisting comorbidities that require management in addition to limb ischemia.

- There are limited high-quality data guiding endovascular or open approaches for the treatment of CTLI. Ongoing trials including BEST-CLI, BASIL-2, and BASIL-3 will hopefully provide additional guidance to this complex problem.

- The selection of open or endovascular therapies for CTLI should weigh patient risk, lesion anatomy, extent of wound, and availability of conduit.

- CDT has a similar limb salvage rate to surgical intervention and is the mainstay of therapy in patients with marginally threatened limbs (Class IIa ischemia).

- Those immediately threatened limbs (Class IIb ischemia) with motor deficits require more rapid restoration of flow with open techniques or endovascular techniques that can establish flow in a single setting.

DISCLOSURE

The author has nothing to disclose.

REFERENCES

1. Norgren L, Hiatt WR, Dormandy JA, et al. Inter-society Consensus for the management of peripheral arterial disease (TASC II). J Vasc Surg 2007; 45(Suppl S):S5–67.

2. Abu Dabrh AM, Steffen MW, Undavalli C, et al. The natural history of untreated severe or critical limb ischemia. J Vasc Surg 2015;62(6):1642–51.e3.

3. Results of a prospective randomized trial evaluating surgery versus thrombolysis for ischemia of the lower extremity. The STILE trial. Ann Surg 1994; 220(3):251–66 [discussion 266-268].

4. Ouriel K, Veith FJ, Sasahara AA. A comparison of recombinant urokinase with vascular surgery as initial treatment for acute arterial occlusion of the legs. Thrombolysis or Peripheral Arterial Surgery (TOPAS) Investigators. N Engl J Med 1998;338(16):1105–11.

5. Ouriel K, Shortell CK, DeWeese JA, et al. A comparison of thrombolytic therapy with operative revascularization in the initial treatment of acute peripheral arterial ischemia. J Vasc Surg 1994;19(6): 1021–30.

6. Menard MT, Farber A. The BEST-CLI trial: a multidisciplinary effort to assess whether surgical or endovascular therapy is better for patients with critical limb ischemia. Semin Vasc Surg 2014;27(1):82–4.

7. Adam DJ, Beard JD, Cleveland T, et al. Bypass versus angioplasty in severe ischaemia of the leg (BASIL): multicentre, randomised controlled trial. Lancet 2005;366(9501):1925–34.

8. Menard MT, Farber A, Assmann SF, et al. Design and rationale of the best endovascular versus best surgical therapy for patients with critical limb ischemia (BEST-CLI) trial. J Am Heart Assoc 2016; 5(7):e003219.

9. Conte MS, Bradbury AW, Kolh P, et al. Global vascular guidelines on the management of chronic limb-threatening ischemia. J Vasc Surg 2019; 69(6S):3S–125S.e40.

10. Gerhard-Herman MD, Gornik HL, Barrett C, et al. 2016 AHA/ACC guideline on the management of patients with lower extremity peripheral artery disease: a report of the American college of cardiology/

American heart association task force on clinical practice guidelines. Circulation 2017;135(12): e726–79.

11. Mills JL, Conte MS, Armstrong DG, et al. The society for vascular surgery lower extremity threatened limb classification system: risk stratification based on wound, ischemia, and foot infection (WIfI). J Vasc Surg 2014;59(1):220–34. e1-2.

12. Darling JD, McCallum JC, Soden PA, et al. Predictive ability of the Society for Vascular Surgery Wound, Ischemia, and foot Infection (WIfI) classification system following infrapopliteal endovascular interventions for critical limb ischemia. J Vasc Surg 2016;64(3):616–22.

13. Robinson WP, Loretz L, Hanesian C, et al. Society for Vascular Surgery Wound, Ischemia, foot Infection (WIfI) score correlates with the intensity of multimodal limb treatment and patient-centered outcomes in patients with threatened limbs managed in a limb preservation center. J Vasc Surg 2017; 66(2):488–98.e2.

14. Popplewell MA, Davies H, Jarrett H, et al. Bypass versus angio plasty in severe ischaemia of the leg - 2 (BASIL-2) trial: study protocol for a randomised controlled trial. Trials 2016;17:11.

15. Simons JP, Schanzer A, Flahive JM, et al. Survival prediction in patients with chronic limb-threatening ischemia who undergo infrainguinal revascularization. J Vasc Surg 2019;69(6S):137S–51S.e3.

16. Biancari F, Salenius J-P, Heikkinen M, et al. Risk-scoring method for prediction of 30-day postoperative outcome after infrainguinal surgical revascularization for critical lower-limb ischemia: a Finnvasc registry study. World J Surg 2007;31(1):217–25 [discussion 226-227].

17. Salaun P, Desormais I, Lapébie F-X, et al. Comparison of ankle pressure, systolic toe pressure, and transcutaneous Oxygen pressure to predict major amputation after 1 year in the COPART cohort. Angiology 2019;70(3):229–36.

18. Schanzer A, Hevelone N, Owens CD, et al. Technical factors affecting autogenous vein graft failure: observations from a large multicenter trial. J Vasc Surg 2007;46(6):1180–90 [discussion 1190].

19. Rzucidlo EM, Powell RJ, Zwolak RM, et al. Early results of stent-grafting to treat diffuse aortoiliac occlusive disease. J Vasc Surg 2003;37(6):1175–80.

20. Jongkind V, Akkersdijk GJM, Yeung KK, et al. A systematic review of endovascular treatment of extensive aortoiliac occlusive disease. J Vasc Surg 2010;52(5):1376–83.

21. Laird JR, Katzen BT, Scheinert D, et al. Nitinol stent implantation vs. Balloon angioplasty for lesions in the superficial femoral and proximal popliteal arteries of patients with claudication: three-year follow-up from the RESILIENT randomized trial. J Endovasc Ther 2012;19(1):1–9.

22. Rosenfield K, Jaff MR, White CJ, et al. Trial of a paclitaxel-coated balloon for femoropopliteal artery disease. N Engl J Med 2015;373(2):145–53.

23. Scheinert D, Duda S, Zeller T, et al. The LEVANT I (Lutonix paclitaxel-coated balloon for the prevention of femoropopliteal restenosis) trial for femoropopliteal revascularization: first-in-human randomized trial of low-dose drug-coated balloon versus uncoated balloon angioplasty. JACC Cardiovasc Interv 2014;7(1):10–9.

24. Tepe G, Schnorr B, Albrecht T, et al. Angioplasty of femoral-popliteal arteries with drug-coated balloons: 5-year follow-up of the THUNDER trial. JACC Cardiovasc Interv 2015;8(1 Pt A):102–8.

25. Bosiers M, Peeters P, Tessarek J, et al. The Zilver® PTX® single arm study: 12-month results from the TASC C/D lesion subgroup. J Cardiovasc Surg (Torino) 2013;54(1):8.

26. Katsanos K, Spiliopoulos S, Kitrou P, et al. Risk of death following application of paclitaxel-coated balloons and stents in the femoropopliteal artery of the leg: a systematic review and meta-analysis of randomized controlled trials. J Am Heart Assoc 2018; 7(24):e011245.

27. Gray WA, Jaff MR, Parikh SA, et al. Mortality assessment of paclitaxel-coated balloons: patient-level meta-analysis of the ILLUMENATE clinical program at 3 years. Circulation 2019;140(14):1145–55.

28. Schneider PA, Varcoe RL, Secemsky E, et al. Update on paclitaxel for femoral-popliteal occlusive disease in the 15 months following a summary level meta-analysis demonstrated increased risk of late mortality and dose response to paclitaxel. J Vasc Surg 2021;73(1):311–22.

29. Rocha-Singh KJ, Beckman JA, Ansel G, et al. Patient-level meta-analysis of 999 claudicants undergoing primary femoropopliteal nitinol stent implantation. Catheter Cardiovasc Interv 2017; 89(7):1250–6.

30. Katsanos K, Spiliopoulos S, Diamantopoulos A, et al. Wound healing outcomes and health-related quality-of-life changes in the ACHILLES trial: 1-year results from a prospective randomized controlled trial of infrapopliteal balloon angioplasty versus sirolimus-eluting stenting in patients with ischemic peripheral arterial disease. JACC Cardiovasc Interv 2016; 9(3):259–67.

31. Scheinert D, Katsanos K, Zeller T, et al. A prospective randomized multicenter comparison of balloon angioplasty and infrapopliteal stenting with the sirolimus-eluting stent in patients with ischemic peripheral arterial disease: 1-year results from the ACHILLES trial. J Am Coll Cardiol 2012; 60(22):2290–5.

32. Zeller T, Baumgartner I, Scheinert D, et al. Drug-eluting balloon versus standard balloon angioplasty for infrapopliteal arterial revascularization in critical

limb ischemia: 12-month results from the IN.PACT DEEP randomized trial. J Am Coll Cardiol 2014; 64(15):1568–76.

33. McKinsey JF, Zeller T, Rocha-Singh KJ, et al. Lower extremity revascularization using directional atherectomy: 12-month prospective results of the DEFINITIVE LE study. JACC Cardiovasc Interv 2014;7(8): 923–33.

34. Söderström M, Albäck A, Biancari F, et al. Angiosome-targeted infrapopliteal endovascular revascularization for treatment of diabetic foot ulcers. J Vasc Surg 2013;57(2):427–35.

35. Settembre N, Biancari F, Spillerova K, et al. Competing risk analysis of the impact of pedal arch status and angiosome-targeted revascularization in chronic limb-threatening ischemia. Ann Vasc Surg 2020;68:384–90.

36. Biancari F, Juvonen T. Angiosome-targeted lower limb revascularization for ischemic foot wounds: systematic review and meta-analysis. Eur J Vasc Endovasc Surg 2014;47(5):517–22.

37. Kum S, Huizing E, Schreve MA, et al. Percutaneous deep venous arterialization in patients with critical limb ischemia. J Cardiovasc Surg (Torino) 2018; 59(5):665–9.

38. Mustapha JA, Saab FA, Clair D, et al. Interim results of the PROMISE I trial to investigate the LimFlow system of percutaneous deep vein arterialization for the treatment of critical limb ischemia. J Invasive Cardiol 2019;31(3):57–63.

39. de Vries SO, Hunink MG. Results of aortic bifurcation grafts for aortoiliac occlusive disease: a meta-analysis. J Vasc Surg 1997;26(4):558–69.

40. Sharma G, Scully RE, Shah SK, et al. Thirty-year trends in aortofemoral bypass for aortoiliac occlusive disease. J Vasc Surg 2018;68(6):1796–804.e2.

41. Siracuse JJ, Gill HL, Schneider DB, et al. Assessing the perioperative safety of common femoral endarterectomy in the endovascular era. Vasc Endovascular Surg 2014;48(1):27–33.

42. Reifsnyder T, Arhuidese IJ, Hicks CW, et al. Contemporary outcomes for open infrainguinal bypass in the endovascular era. Ann Vasc Surg 2016;30:52–8.

43. Eugster T, Stierli P, Guerke L, et al. Present status of infrainguinal arterial bypass procedures following an all autogenous policy–long-term results of a single center. Swiss Surg 2002;8(4):171–5.

44. Goshima KR, Mills JL, Hughes JD. A new look at outcomes after infrainguinal bypass surgery: traditional reporting standards systematically underestimate the expenditure of effort required to attain limb salvage. J Vasc Surg 2004;39(2):330–5.

45. Bradbury AW, Adam DJ, Bell J, et al. Multicentre randomised controlled trial of the clinical and cost-effectiveness of a bypass-surgery-first versus a balloon-angioplasty-first revascularisation strategy for severe limb ischaemia due to infrainguinal disease. The Bypass versus Angioplasty in Severe Ischaemia of the Leg (BASIL) trial. Health Technol Assess 2010;14(14):1–210. iii-iv.

46. Bradbury AW, Adam DJ, Bell J, et al. Bypass versus Angioplasty in Severe Ischaemia of the Leg (BASIL) trial: an intention-to-treat analysis of amputation-free and overall survival in patients randomized to a bypass surgery-first or a balloon angioplasty-first revascularization strategy. J Vasc Surg 2010;51(5): 5S–17S.

47. Bradbury AW, Adam DJ, Bell J, et al. Bypass versus Angioplasty in Severe Ischaemia of the Leg (BASIL) trial: analysis of amputation free and overall survival by treatment received. J Vasc Surg 2010;51(5 Suppl):18S–31S.

48. Peters CML, de Vries J, Lodder P, et al. Quality of life and not health status improves after major amputation in the elderly critical limb ischaemia patient. Eur J Vasc Endovasc Surg 2019;57(4):547–53.

49. Writing Committee Members, Creager MA, Belkin M, et al. 2012 ACCF/AHA/ACR/SCAI/SIR/STS/SVM/ SVN/SVS key data elements and definitions for peripheral atherosclerotic vascular disease: a report of the American College of Cardiology Foundation/ American Heart Association task force on clinical data standards (writing committee to develop clinical data standards for peripheral atherosclerotic vascular disease). Circulation 2012;125(2):395–467.

50. Creager MA, Kaufman JA, Conte MS. Acute limb ischemia. N Engl J Med 2012;366(23):2198–206.

51. Duval S, Keo HH, Oldenburg NC, et al. The impact of prolonged lower limb ischemia on amputation, mortality, and functional status: the FRIENDS registry. Am Heart J 2014;168(4):577–87.

52. Bekwelem W, Connolly SJ, Halperin JL, et al. Extracranial systemic embolic events in patients with non-valvular atrial fibrillation: incidence, risk factors, and outcomes. Circulation 2015;132(9):796–803.

53. Rutherford RB, Baker JD, Ernst C, et al. Recommended standards for reports dealing with lower extremity ischemia: revised version. J Vasc Surg 1997; 26(3):517–38.

54. Theodoridis PG, Davos CH, Dodos I, et al. Thrombolysis in acute lower limb ischemia: review of the current literature. Ann Vasc Surg 2018;52:255–62.

55. Schrijver A, Vos J, Hoksbergen AW, et al. Ultrasound-accelerated thrombolysis for lower extremity ischemia: multicenter experience and literature review. J Cardiovasc Surg (Torino) 2011;52(4):467–76.

56. Lopez R, Yamashita TS, Neisen M, et al. Single-center experience with Indigo aspiration thrombectomy for acute lower limb ischemia. J Vasc Surg 2020; 72(1):226–32.

57. Ansel GM, Botti CF, Silver MJ. Treatment of acute limb ischemia with a percutaneous mechanical thrombectomy-based endovascular approach: 5-year limb salvage and survival results from a single

center series. Catheter Cardiovasc Interv 2008; 72(3):325–30.

58. Silva JA, Ramee SR, Collins TJ, et al. Rheolytic thrombectomy in the treatment of acute limb-threatening ischemia: immediate results and six-month follow-up of the multicenter AngioJet registry. Possis Peripheral AngioJet Study AngioJet Investigators. Cathet Cardiovasc Diagn 1998;45(4): 386–93.

59. Fogarty TJ, Cranley JJ, Krause RJ, et al. A method for extraction of arterial emboli and thrombi. Surg Gynecol Obstet 1963;116:241–4.

60. Campbell WB, Marriott S, Eve R, et al. Amputation for acute ischaemia is associated with increased co-morbidity and higher amputation level. Cardiovasc Surg 2003;11(2):121–3.

61. Kuukasjärvi P, Salenius JP. Perioperative outcome of acute lower limb ischaemia on the basis of the national vascular registry. The Finnvasc Study Group. Eur J Vasc Surg 1994;8(5):578–83.

62. Campbell WB, Ridler BM, Szymanska TH. Current management of acute leg ischaemia: results of an audit by the Vascular Surgical Society of Great Britain and Ireland. Br J Surg 1998;85(11):1498–503.

Acute Aortic Syndromes

R. Kevin Rogers, MD, MSc[a],*, T. Brett Reece, MD[b], Marc P. Bonaca, MD, MPH[a,c],
Connie N. Hess, MD, MHS[a,c]

KEYWORDS

- Acute aortic syndrome • Aortic dissection • Intramural hematoma • Penetrating aortic ulcer

KEY POINTS

- Acute aortic syndromes are composed of aortic dissection (80%–90%), intramural hematoma, and penetrating aortic ulcers.
- Rapid diagnosis is essential to optimize patient outcomes. It is facilitated by heightened provider awareness in patients with both characteristic pain and nonspecific symptoms with risk factors for dissection.
- Electrocardiogram-gated computed tomography angiography of the chest, abdomen, and pelvis is the most practical imaging modality for diagnosis and identification of complications.
- Adjunctive echocardiography is used to identify aortic valve pathology.
- Emergent surgery is indicated for acute aortic syndromes involving the ascending aorta. Developments in surgical techniques are improving patient outcomes.
- Evolving endovascular techniques for acute aortic syndromes limited to the descending thoracic aorta are complementary to optimal medical therapy.

 Video content accompanies this article at http://www.cardiology.theclinics.com.

BACKGROUND AND CLINICAL SIGNIFICANCE

The first description of an acute aortic syndrome was in 1760 from the autopsy of King George II.[1,2] Nearly 200 years later, the first successful surgery for an aortic dissection was published by DeBakey and colleagues.[3] In the 1990s, the development of the International Registry of Acute Aortic Dissections (IRAD) has advanced the knowledge base around acute aortic syndromes, and the introduction of aortic endografts has expanded therapeutic options.[4]

Acute aortic syndromes include aortic dissection (80%–90% of acute aortic syndromes), intramural hematoma (IMH), and penetrating aortic ulcer (PAU).[5] The incidence of acute aortic syndromes is 3.5 to 6.0 per 100,000 patient-years, and contemporary in-hospital mortality rate for acute aortic syndromes derived from the IRAD registry is ∼21%. In comparison, the incidence of acute myocardial infarction in the United States is approximately 40-fold higher,[6–8] yet in-hospital mortality is 5 times lower than that for acute aortic syndromes.[9,10]

Although acute aortic syndromes are not the most prevalent cardiovascular disease, they portend high patient mortality and contribute to increased costs for health care systems. On average, hospitalization is 14 days for patients with acute aortic syndromes, and total hospital costs in Canada in 2017 approached $21 million Canadian dollars (equivalent to $16 million US dollars).[4,11] Prompt diagnosis and optimal management are imperative to yield the most favorable patient outcomes.[12,13] Herein, the authors review

[a] Division of Cardiology, University of Colorado, School of Medicine, Section of Vascular Medicine, Mail Stop B132, Leprino Building, 12401 East 17th Avenue, Room 560, Aurora, CO 80045, USA; [b] Division of Cardiovascular Surgery, University of Colorado, School of Medicine, 12631 East 17th Avenue, Room 6111, Aurora, CO 80045, USA; [c] CPC Clinical Research, 2115 North Scranton Street Suite 2040, Aurora, CO 80045, USA
* Corresponding author.
E-mail address: Kevin.Rogers@cuanschutz.edu

Cardiol Clin 39 (2021) 495–503
https://doi.org/10.1016/j.ccl.2021.06.002

the definition, clinical presentation, diagnosis, and management of acute aortic syndromes.

DEFINITIONS

Acute aortic syndromes can be classified into aortic dissection, IMH, and PAU. An acute aortic dissection involves an intimal defect that leads to bleeding into the media of the aorta followed by the creation of a dissection plane separating a false lumen within the aortic wall and the true lumen of the aorta.[14] An intramural hematoma is characterized by bleeding or thrombus formation within the aortic media without an obvious intimal defect.[15] In contrast, a PAU is defined as a clear intimal defect of atherosclerotic aortic plaque with communication of blood to the aortic media, which can be a nidus of blood flow into a false lumen plane (**Fig. 1**).[16]

Because the anatomic location of acute aortic pathology often drives management, knowledge of aortic anatomy is important. The aorta consists of the aortic root, ascending aorta, aortic arch, descending aorta, and abdominal aorta (**Fig. 2**). Two well-known anatomic descriptions of aortic dissection exist—the Stanford and DeBakey classifications—which focus on the involvement of the ascending aorta and aortic arch branch vessels[14,16] (**Fig. 3**). In general, acute aortic syndromes affecting the ascending thoracic aorta (Stanford A, Debakey 1 and 2) mandate emergent surgery, whereas descending thoracic aortic pathology propagating distally to the abdominal aortic branch vessels risk malperfusion syndromes, which complicate management and increase mortality.[17] In addition, acute aortic dissections affecting the aortic root may necessitate aortic valve replacement and coronary artery revascularization.

CLINICAL PRESENTATION AND DIAGNOSIS

Acute aortic syndromes often present with a variety of symptoms and complications, including acute myocardial infarction, acute aortic regurgitation, pericardial tamponade, and more distal rupture, as well as ischemia of the extremities, viscera, and central nervous system. The initial history, physical examination, and imaging modalities are directed to diagnose an acute aortic syndrome and identify its complications.

There is not a single clinical profile for the patient presenting with an acute aortic syndrome. In a systematic review of acute aortic dissection encompassing 82 studies and 57,311 patients, presenting patients had a median age of 61 years, were more often men (50%–81% across studies),

and had hypertension as the most common risk factor followed by smoking.[7] Patients with genetic predispositions such as Marfan (5% in IRAD), vascular Ehlers Danlos, Turner syndrome, and Loeys-Dietz syndromes may present without other typical risk factors and at an earlier age.[6,18]

Symptoms and Signs

Pain is the most common and important presenting symptom in patients with acute aortic syndromes. In a report of the first 2000 patients from IRAD, the sudden onset of severe pain was recorded in 85% of patients.[18] The majority reported pain in the chest, although patients with type B dissections frequently reported pain in the abdomen or back.[18] The quality of the pain is abrupt and "sharp" or "tearing," in contrast to the discomfort experienced in acute myocardial infarction.[18] A small minority of patients (6.4%) presented with a painless aortic dissection.[18] A high index of suspicion for acute aortic dissection is necessary in patients presenting with sudden chest, abdominal, or back pain, especially in the presence of syncope, hypotension, or evidence of cerebral, visceral, or extremity malperfusion. For the patient with syncope and/or hypotension (30% of patients in IRAD), the physical examination should include auscultation for the murmur of acute aortic insufficiency and evaluation for potential cardiac tamponade (pulsus paradoxus and jugular venous pulse assessment). A complete pulse and neurologic examination is important to identify objective evidence of ischemia: in IRAD, 30% of patients exhibited a pulse deficit.[18] The history and physical examination can then catalyze appropriate imaging to confirm the diagnosis of an acute aortic syndrome and identify its complications.

Biomarkers

Serologic biomarkers are attractive conceptually to aid in the initial evaluation of an acute aortic syndrome, which can be missed in up to 40% of cases due to nonspecific presenting signs and symptoms.[12] Because acute aortic syndromes involve damage to the aortic media, components of the media, as well as markers of thrombosis and inflammation, have been a focus for identifying clinically useful biomarkers (**Table 1**).[13] D-dimer is the most studied potential biomarker, as a readily available assay exists, but levels are also elevated in a competing potential diagnosis in the patient with chest pain, namely pulmonary embolism. Unfortunately, widespread clinical utility of serologic biomarkers for diagnosing acute aortic syndromes has remained low due to a variety of

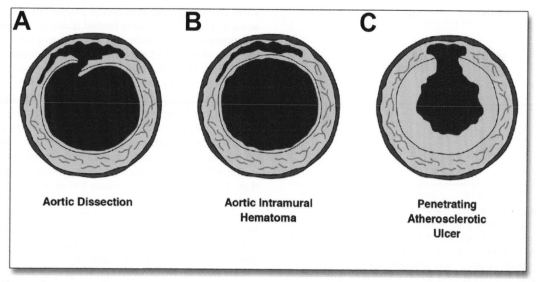

A   **B**   **C**

Aortic Dissection   **Aortic Intramural Hematoma**   **Penetrating Atherosclerotic Ulcer**

Fig. 1. Three types of acute aortic syndromes. (*A*) Aortic dissection. (*B*) Intramural hematoma. (*C*) Penetrating aortic ulcer. (*From* Baliga RR, Nienaber CA, Bossone E, Oh JK, Isselbacher EM, Sechtem U, Fattori R, Raman SV and Eagle KA. The role of imaging in aortic dissection and related syndromes. *JACC Cardiovasc Imaging.* 2014;7:406-24; with permission.)

limitations, including lack of point-of-care assays, rapid decrease in levels following the inciting event, and poor diagnostic performance.[13,14]

Imaging

Imaging modalities for acute aortic syndromes include computed tomography (CT), echocardiography, MRI, and chest radiograph. Practically, diagnosis and assessment of complications from an acute aortic dissection is readily achieved with an

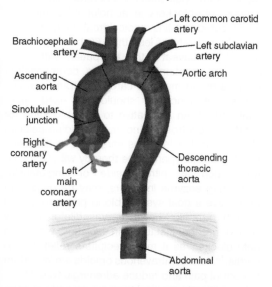

Left common carotid artery
Brachiocephalic artery
Left subclavian artery
Ascending aorta
Aortic arch
Sinotubular junction
Right coronary artery
Left main coronary artery
Descending thoracic aorta
Abdominal aorta

Fig. 2. Anatomy of the thoracic and abdominal aorta. (*From* Taylor AJ. Atlas of cardiovascular computed tomography: an imaging companion to Braunwald's heart disease, Philadelphia, 2010, Elsevier.)

electrocardiogram (ECG)-gated CT angiogram and transthoracic echocardiography. An electrocardiogram is also important to evaluate alternative causes of chest pain and identify coronary malperfusion, often involving the right coronary artery, for patients with a Stanford type A dissection.

The chest radiograph is often an initial test for the patient with chest pain, but the classic finding of a widened mediastinum is absent in up to 28% of cases.[7,14,16] As such, the chest radiograph is not sufficient to exclude an acute aortic syndrome when clinical suspicion is present.

CT angiography is the preferred imaging modality for acute aortic syndromes in most situations (**Fig. 4**).[5] Its diagnostic performance is excellent, with sensitivity of 95% to 100% and specificity of 98% to 100% for aortic dissection.[5,7] ECG-gated CT angiography is also able to identify involvement of the coronary artery ostia and pathology of the aortic valve. Furthermore, CT angiography can image the entire thoracic and abdominal aorta, characterize the true and false lumen of a dissection, and identify which lumen supplies major branch vessels.[5] CT is widely available and provides rapid clinical data. Disadvantages of CT include exposure to ionizing radiation and complications from administration of iodinated contrast (nephropathy and hypersensitivity reactions).[5] These disadvantages are usually outweighed by the benefit of rapid and accurate diagnosis of an acute aortic syndrome.

Transthoracic echocardiography (TTE) is inferior to CT in its diagnostic performance for acute aortic syndromes, with sensitivities and specificities as

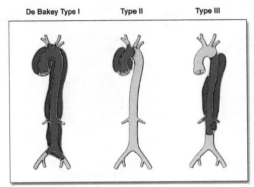

Fig. 3. Anatomic classifications of aortic dissection. The *DeBakey classification* focuses on the location of the intimal defect and the extent of the dissection. A DeBakey type 1 dissection originates in the ascending aorta but involves the aortic arch and even the descending aorta. A DeBakey type II dissection is confined to the ascending aorta. A DeBakey type III dissection is limited to the descending thoracic aorta, perhaps extending into the abdominal aorta. The *Stanford classification* focuses on the involvement of the ascending aorta. Stanford type A dissections are localized to the ascending aorta. Stanford type B dissections do not involve the ascending aorta but may affect the aortic arch. (*From* Baliga RR, Nienaber CA, Bossone E, Oh JK, Isselbacher EM, Sechtem U, Fattori R, Raman SV and Eagle KA. The role of imaging in aortic dissection and related syndromes. *JACC Cardiovasc Imaging.* 2014;7:406-24; with permission.)

low as 60% for Stanford type A dissections and even lower for type B dissections.[5,7] However, TTE is a clinically useful adjunctive test for acute aortic dissection. It is readily available, provides rapid results, and can be performed at the bedside. TTE can visualize the proximal 8 mm of the ascending aorta and can identify aortic regurgitation, pericardial effusions, and wall motion abnormalities that might suggest coronary artery involvement.[5] A major limitation of TTE is the inability to visualize the aortic arch and the descending thoracic aorta comprehensively. Thus, although TTE cannot exclude aortic dissection, it as an important imaging modality in patients with acute aortic syndromes to identify complications such as aortic regurgitation and cardiac tamponade.[5]

Transesophageal echocardiography (TEE) has excellent diagnostic performance for acute aortic syndromes. The sensitivity of TEE for acute aortic dissection is approximately 89% and the specificity close to 99%.[5–7,16,19] It can be performed at the bedside and intraoperatively during aortic repair.[14] Other advantages include lack of iodinated contrast and ionizing radiation, provision of results rapidly, and the ability to identify aortic

valve pathology and tamponade physiology. Disadvantages of TEE include limited ability to image the proximal aortic arch and inability to characterize involvement of abdominal aortic branches.[5]

MRI has attractive diagnostic performance for acute aortic dissection with a sensitivity of 95% to 98% and specificity of 94% to 98%.[5,20] Advantages of magnetic resonance (MR) angiography include characterization of aortic insufficiency and the true and false lumens of a dissection flap as well as aortic branch vessel involvement.[5] No iodinated contrast is required nor is ionized radiation. These attributes also make MR angiography attractive for surveillance following aortic repair.[5,6] However, acquisition times are longer for MR than for other imaging modalities, which is impractical in the unstable patient.[6] Another disadvantage of MR is lack of widespread availability.

Intravascular ultrasound is an imaging technique that can guide aortic repair[6] **Fig. 5**). Catheter-based angiography is limited by invasiveness, need for iodinated contrast and ionizing radiation, and less attractive diagnostic performance as compared with CT, MR, and TEE.[14] It is typically reserved for the patient misdiagnosed as having an acute coronary syndrome due to a ruptured atherosclerotic plaque (Video 1).

MANAGEMENT

Regardless of whether a patient with an acute aortic syndrome is managed invasively, medical therapy ("antiimpulse" therapy) is indicated to reduce aortic wall stress and control pain.[14] Intravenous beta-blockers (ie, esmolol or labetalol) are an accepted first-line medical treatment, targeting a goal heart rate of less than 60 beats per minute.[6,14,16] A caveat is that the patient with acute aortic regurgitation may require compensatory tachycardia to maintain cardiac output, in which cases beta-blockade should be used more cautiously.[14] An alternative to beta-blockade for heart rate control is a nonhydropyridine calcium channel blocker, such as verapamil or diltiazem. Additional antihypertensive therapy with vasodilators, such as nitroprusside or angiotensin-converting enzyme inhibitors, may be necessary to achieve a goal systolic blood pressure of 100 to 120 mm Hg; however, vasodilator therapy should not be instituted in isolation without a beta-blocker, as it may precipitate reflex tachycardia.[14] Finally, intravenous opioids are important to control pain and reduce adrenergic tone.[14]

In addition to medical therapy, procedural intervention is frequently indicated, depending on the anatomy of acute aortic pathology and complications. In general, there are few randomized trials

Table 1
Potential serologic biomarkers for acute aortic syndromes

Potential Biomarker	Rationale for Utility	Comments and Limitations
Smooth muscle myosin	Component of vascular smooth muscle	Levels rapidly decrease in first 24 h after AAD
Calponin MMP 8 Tenascin-C	Present in aortic media interstitium	Poor positive predictive value (calponin)
Soluble elastin fragments	Component of elastic laminae	Reduced diagnostic performance with false lumen thrombosis
D-dimer	Fibrin-degradation product and marker of thrombosis	Good sensitivity but lack of specificity

Abbreviation: AAD, acute aortic dissection.

(*Data from* Ranasinghe AM and Bonser RS. Biomarkers in acute aortic dissection and other aortic syndromes. *J Am Coll Cardiol.* 2010;56:1535-41 and Erbel R, Aboyans V, Boileau C, Bossone E, Bartolomeo RD, Eggebrecht H, Evangelista A, Falk V, Frank H, Gaemperli O, Grabenwoger M, Haverich A, Iung B, Manolis AJ, Meijboom F, Nienaber CA, Roffi M, Rousseau H, Sechtem U, Sirnes PA, Allmen RS, Vrints CJ and Guidelines ESCCfP. 2014 ESC Guidelines on the diagnosis and treatment of aortic diseases: Document covering acute and chronic aortic diseases of the thoracic and abdominal aorta of the adult. The Task Force for the Diagnosis and Treatment of Aortic Diseases of the European Society of Cardiology (ESC). *Eur Heart J.* 2014;35:2873-926.)

of management strategies for acute aortic syndromes, and most of the available randomized data are for treatment of type B dissections.

Stanford Type A Acute Aortic Dissection

Surgery is the definitive treatment of type A acute aortic dissections.[6,14,16] In 2952 patients with type A acute aortic dissection enrolled over a 17-year period (1996–2013) in the IRAD registry, the mortality for patients treated medically without surgery was 57%, and the mortality rate remained relatively stable throughout the 17-year period.[9] The proportion of patients treated with surgery increased from 78% at the beginning; this time span to 90% at the end (P<.001).[9] Surgical mortality was observed to be less than that for patients treated medically (25% in the earlier years compared with 18% at the end of the time period, P = .003).[9]

Insights into the reasons for improved surgical mortality over time can be gleaned from a retrospective review of 806 patients who underwent surgical repair of acute aortic dissections at Stanford from 2000 to 2019.[4] In this analysis, 1-year mortality was more favorable in patients treated during 2010 to 2019 as compared with those undergoing surgery from 2000 to 2009 (12% vs 18%, P = .014). The following factors may help to explain the observed temporal trends in improved survival: increased provider awareness, improved imaging with CT angiography, more aggressive repair of the aortic root with or without aortic valve replacement, more extensive aortic arch repair, and increased use of antegrade cerebral perfusion for intraoperative cerebral protection.

Stanford Type B Aortic Dissection

In 1476 patients with type B acute aortic dissection enrolled over a 17-year period (1996–2013) in the IRAD registry, the majority were managed medically (63%) but with trends of increased endovascular treatment rather than medical therapy alone or rather than open surgery over time.[9] The decision to pursue invasive treatment often is dictated by whether type B dissections are "uncomplicated" or "complicated." A "complicated" type B dissection involves ongoing pain, aortic expansion, malperfusion, or signs of rupture.[16]

Uncomplicated type B dissections traditionally were treated noninvasively because the observed mortality for medically treated patients was 10% at 30 days compared with the higher in-hospital mortality with open surgery (approaching 30%).[7,16,21] However, with the emergence of endovascular stent grafts, management strategies of medical therapy alone versus endovascular therapy is now a matter of debate. In the ADSORB trial, 61 patients with uncomplicated type B dissection were randomized to best medical treatment alone or to endovascular stent grafting.[21] The primary outcome was incomplete false lumen thrombosis, aortic dilatation, or aortic rupture at 1 year, which favored the endovascular therapy group[21] (50% of the endovascular therapy group vs 100% of the medical therapy–alone group reached an aortic endpoint, P<.001). In the INSTEAD trial (The INvestigation of STEnt Grafts

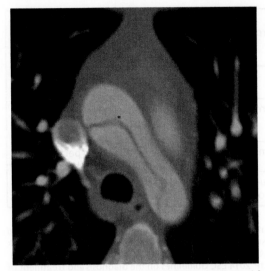

Fig. 4. Axial image of the aortic arch in a patient with acute aortic dissection. *Dissection flap.

in Aortic Dissection), 140 patients with uncomplicated type B dissections (at least 2 weeks following presentation) from 7 European centers were randomized to endovascular therapy plus optimal medical therapy versus optimal medical therapy alone. The trial did not show a difference in the primary outcome of all-cause mortality at 2 years (2-year survival rate of 95.6 ± 2.5% with optimal medical therapy vs 88.9 ± 3.7% with endovascular treatment, $P = .15$). A secondary outcome—aortic-related deaths—was also similar between groups. However, markers of long-term aortic remodeling were more favorable for the stent graft group.[22,23] Until additional randomized

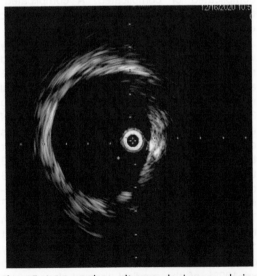

Fig. 5. Intravascular ultrasound image during ascending aortic repair in a patient with acute aortic dissection. *Dissection flap.

trials are conducted, a multidisciplinary approach to intervention with careful evaluation of patient and anatomic and procedural considerations is needed.

"Complicated" type B dissections often require more emergent, invasive treatment. In particular, malperfusion syndromes involve end-organ ischemia (brain, viscera, spine, or extremities) due to dynamic or static obstruction of an aortic branch vessel by the dissection flap.[17] Malperfusion can complicate up to 40% of aortic dissections and portends increased morbidity and mortality.[17] In addition to optimal medical therapy, invasive treatment options include proximal aortic dissection repair, which pressurizes the true lumen, thoracic endovascular aortic repair to cover the primary intimal tear and direct blood flow to the true lumen, endovascular fenestration techniques to pressurize both true and false lumens, and even branch vessel stenting to improve end organ perfusion.[17,24]

Meticulous clinical surveillance is critical to identify patients with developing or ongoing malperfusion that will require invasive treatment. Frequent assessment of new or existing pain syndromes, neurologic examinations, and pulse assessments are mandatory. Unheralded hypertension might be a predictor of renal infarction. Increasing abdominal pain and serum lactate can indicate evolving mesenteric ischemia. Aggressive use of CT angiography can confirm these clinical findings as well as identify propagating dissection and aortic branch compromise.

Intramural Hematoma

IMH comprises a minority of acute aortic syndromes (5%–18%), is localized to the ascending aorta or aortic arch in up to 40% of cases, and is confined to the descending aorta in approximately 60% of cases.[6,15,16] Overall, the reported prognosis of IMH is more favorable than that for acute aortic dissection. However, the natural history of IMH is unpredictable, as 16% to 47% of IMH involving the ascending aorta can progress to acute aortic dissection, particularly if in close proximity to the aortic valve, and should be considered for urgent surgery.[6,7,16] IMH localized to the descending aorta has a more favorable prognosis, similar to uncomplicated type B dissections, and can be treated conservatively with heart rate and blood pressure control and imaging surveillance.[7,16]

Penetrating Aortic Ulcer

PAU comprise even a smaller minority of acute aortic syndromes (2%–7%) and are limited to

Table 2
Aortic surgeries

Anatomic Segment	Type of Surgery	Description/Comments
Aortic Root	Aortic valve resuspension	Performed if normal aortic diameter free of intimal defect but aortic valve pathology is present
	Aortic valve replacement	Performed if aortic pathology is present but aortic root is otherwise normal
	Valve-sparing root	Performed if aortic root is involved but aortic leaflets function normally
Coronary Arteries	Cabrol/HemiCabrol	Side-to-side anastomosis of coronary arteries to ascending aortic interposition graft
	Reimplantation with coronary "button"	End-to-side anastomosis of coronary arteries to ascending aortic interposition graft
	Supracoronary bypass	Traditional coronary artery bypass grafting
Ascending Aorta	Ascending aorta replacement	If no involvement of the arch, the aorta is clamped just proximal to the innominate. If the arch is affected, an open distal anastomosis is performed
Aortic Arch	Hemi-arch repair	The inferior portion of the arch is replaced, preserving the origins of the great vessels
	Bypass of the great vessels	The arch is replaced with bypass of 1 or more of the great vessels
	Total arch replacement	The entire aortic arch is replaced with end-to-end anastomoses of the graft to the great vessels
	"Frozen elephant trunk"	Hybrid prosthesis is used to reimplant the great arch vessels and place an endograft in the descending thoracic aorta if it is also diseased
Descending Aorta and/or Abdominal Aorta	Open repair	The descending and/or abdominal aorta is repaired with an open surgical procedure
	Stent graft	A self-expanding endovascular stent is placed to repair the descending thoracic and/or abdominal aorta
	Fenestration	Angioplasty and stenting of the dissection flap joining true and false lumens

the descending thoracic aorta in 90% of cases.[6,14,16] The natural history is unclear.[6] Because the anatomic location of PAU is typically limited to the descending aorta, close clinical surveillance for recurrent pain and imaging surveillance, with CT or MR angiography, is the initial management approach.[6,16] Invasive treatment can usually be performed with an endovascular stent graft and is reserved for refractory pain, signs of contained rupture, rapid increase in the depth of the ulcer, or a 1-cm width and depth of the ulcer[16] (**Table 2**).

SUMMARY

Acute aortic syndromes portend high early mortality and substantial morbidity. Patients with acute aortic syndromes often present with nonspecific clinical symptoms and signs. Thus, it is important for providers to maintain a high index of suspicion for acute aortic syndromes. CT angiography and echocardiography are rapid, useful imaging modalities to diagnose acute aortic syndromes and identify complications. Emergent surgery is indicated for acute aortic syndromes involving the ascending aorta and aortic branch vessels. Emergent surgery or endovascular intervention is also indicated for thoracoabdominal acute aortic syndromes when there is end-organ malperfusion. Optimal medical therapy alone is appropriate for uncomplicated acute aortic syndromes involving the descending aorta. Organizing multidisciplinary "aortic teams" within health care systems should be explored to increase the speed of diagnosis and maximize patient outcomes. Finally, randomized trials in patients with acute aortic syndromes would be beneficial to guide management strategies but will be difficult to conduct in this population.

CLINICS CARE POINTS

- Acute aortic syndromes include aortic dissection (80%–90% of acute aortic syndromes), intramural hematoma (IMH), and penetrating aortic ulcer (PAU).

- In general, acute aortic syndromes affecting the ascending thoracic aorta (Stanford A, Debakey 1 and 2) mandate emergent surgery, whereas descending thoracic aortic pathology propagating distally to the abdominal aortic branch vessels risk malperfusion syndromes, which complicate management and increase mortality.

- Acute aortic syndromes often present with a variety of symptoms and complications, including acute myocardial infarction, acute aortic regurgitation, pericardial tamponade, and more distal rupture, as well as ischemia of the extremities, viscera, and central nervous system.

- CT angiography is the preferred imaging modality for acute aortic syndromes.

- Regardless of whether a patient with an acute aortic syndrome is managed invasively, medical therapy ("antiimpulse" therapy) is indicated to reduce aortic wall stress and control pain.

- Surgery is the definitive treatment of type A acute aortic dissections.

- The decision to pursue invasive treatment often is dictated by whether type B dissections are "uncomplicated" or "complicated." A "complicated" type B dissection involves ongoing pain, aortic expansion, malperfusion, or signs of rupture.

- IMH comprises a minority of acute aortic syndromes (5%–18%), is localized to the ascending aorta or aortic arch in up to 40% of cases, and is confined to the descending aorta in approximately 60% of cases.

DISCLOSURE

The authors have nothing to disclose.

SUPPLEMENTARY DATA

Supplementary data to this article can be found online at https://doi.org/10.1016/j.ccl.2021.06.002.

REFERENCES

1. Corvera JS. Acute aortic syndrome. Ann Cardiothorac Surg 2016;5:188–93.
2. Criado FJ. Aortic dissection: a 250-year perspective. Tex Heart Inst J 2011;38:694–700.
3. De Bakey ME, Cooley DA, Creech O Jr. Surgical considerations of dissecting aneurysm of the aorta. Ann Surg 1955;142:586–610. discussion, 611-2.
4. Zhu Y, Lingala B, Baiocchi M, et al. Type A aortic dissection-experience over 5 decades: JACC historical breakthroughs in perspective. J Am Coll Cardiol 2020;76:1703–13.
5. Baliga RR, Nienaber CA, Bossone E, et al. The role of imaging in aortic dissection and related syndromes. JACC Cardiovasc Imaging 2014;7:406–24.
6. Bossone E, LaBounty TM, Eagle KA. Acute aortic syndromes: diagnosis and management, an update. Eur Heart J 2018;39:739–749d.
7. Mussa FF, Horton JD, Moridzadeh R, et al. Acute aortic dissection and intramural hematoma: a systematic review. JAMA 2016;316:754–63.
8. Reynolds K, Go AS, Leong TK, et al. Trends in incidence of hospitalized acute myocardial infarction in the Cardiovascular Research Network (CVRN). Am J Med 2017;130:317–27.
9. Pape LA, Awais M, Woznicki EM, et al. Presentation, diagnosis, and outcomes of acute aortic dissection: 17-year trends from the International Registry of Acute Aortic Dissection. J Am Coll Cardiol 2015;66:350–8.
10. McNamara RL, Kennedy KF, Cohen DJ, et al. Predicting in-hospital mortality in patients with acute

myocardial infarction. J Am Coll Cardiol 2016;68: 626–35.

11. McClure RS, Brogly SB, Lajkosz K, et al. Economic burden and healthcare resource use for thoracic aortic dissections and thoracic aortic aneurysms-a population-based cost-of-illness analysis. J Am Heart Assoc 2020;9:e014981.

12. Olin JW, Fuster V. Acute aortic dissection: the need for rapid, accurate, and readily available diagnostic strategies. Arterioscler Thromb Vasc Biol 2003;23:1721–3.

13. Ranasinghe AM, Bonser RS. Biomarkers in acute aortic dissection and other aortic syndromes. J Am Coll Cardiol 2010;56:1535–41.

14. Hiratzka LF, Bakris GL, Beckman JA, et al, American College of Cardiology F, American Heart Association Task Force on Practice G, American Association for Thoracic S, American College of R, American Stroke A, Society of Cardiovascular A, Society for Cardiovascular A, Interventions, Society of Interventional R, Society of Thoracic S and Society for Vascular M. 2010 ACCF/AHA/AATS/ACR/ASA/SCA/SCAI/ SIR/STS/SVM guidelines for the diagnosis and management of patients with thoracic aortic disease: executive summary. A report of the American College of Cardiology Foundation/American Heart Association Task Force on Practice Guidelines, American Association for Thoracic Surgery, American College of Radiology, American Stroke Association, Society of Cardiovascular Anesthesiologists, Society for Cardiovascular Angiography and Interventions, Society of Interventional Radiology, Society of Thoracic Surgeons, and Society for Vascular Medicine. Catheter Cardiovasc Interv 2010;76:E43–86.

15. Al Rstum Z, Tanaka A, Eisenberg SB, et al. Optimal timing of type A intramural hematoma repair. Ann Cardiothorac Surg 2019;8:524–30.

16. Erbel R, Aboyans V, Boileau C, et al, Guidelines ESCCfP. 2014 ESC Guidelines on the diagnosis and treatment of aortic diseases: Document covering acute and chronic aortic diseases of the thoracic and abdominal aorta of the adult. The Task Force for the Diagnosis and Treatment of Aortic Diseases of the European Society of Cardiology (ESC). Eur Heart J 2014;35:2873–926.

17. Norton EL, Khaja MS, Williams DM, et al. Type A aortic dissection complicated by malperfusion syndrome. Curr Opin Cardiol 2019;34:610–5.

18. Tsai TT, Trimarchi S, Nienaber CA. Acute aortic dissection: perspectives from the International registry of acute aortic dissection (IRAD). Eur J Vasc Endovasc Surg 2009;37:149–59.

19. Bossone E, Evangelista A, Isselbacher E, et al, International Registry of Acute Aortic Dissection I. Prognostic role of transesophageal echocardiography in acute type A aortic dissection. Am Heart J 2007;153: 1013–20.

20. Shiga T, Wajima Z, Apfel CC, et al. Diagnostic accuracy of transesophageal echocardiography, helical computed tomography, and magnetic resonance imaging for suspected thoracic aortic dissection: systematic review and meta-analysis. Arch Intern Med 2006;166:1350–6.

21. Brunkwall J, Kasprzak P, Verhoeven E, et al. Endovascular repair of acute uncomplicated aortic type B dissection promotes aortic remodelling: 1 year results of the ADSORB trial. Eur J Vasc Endovasc Surg 2014;48:285–91.

22. Nienaber CA, Rousseau H, Eggebrecht H, et al. Randomized comparison of strategies for type B aortic dissection: the INvestigation of STEnt Grafts in Aortic Dissection (INSTEAD) trial. Circulation 2009;120:2519–28.

23. Nienaber CA, Kische S, Rousseau H, et al. Endovascular repair of type B aortic dissection: long-term results of the randomized investigation of stent grafts in aortic dissection trial. Circ Cardiovasc Interv 2013;6:407–16.

24. Yang B, Patel HJ, Williams DM, et al. Management of type A dissection with malperfusion. Ann Cardiothorac Surg 2016;5:265–74.

Thoracic Aortic Aneurysm
A Clinical Review

Ethan M. Senser, MD[a], Shantum Misra, MD[b], Stanislav Henkin, MD, MPH[a],*

KEYWORDS

- Thoracic aortic aneurysm • Thoracic aortic dissection • Marfan syndrome • Loeys-Dietz syndrome
- Vascular Ehlers-Danlos syndrome • Bicuspid aortic valve

KEY POINTS

- In the United States, in 2018, almost 10,000 deaths were attributed to aortic aneurysms.
- Over 95% of thoracic aortic aneurysms are asymptomatic until the point of dissection or rupture. Majority of aneurysms are discovered incidentally.
- Initial aneurysm size at the time of diagnosis is the best predictor of growth rate and subsequent risk of rupture, but family history, genetics, coexistent hypertension, and smoking can adversely impact the natural history of TAA.
- Surveillance imaging and referral for prophylactic surgical aortic repair based on absolute diameter and individual genetic, familial, and syndromic risk factors is the primary means to decrease mortality from thoracic aortic aneurysm.

INTRODUCTION

Thoracic aortic aneurysms (TAA) are a common clinical entity seen in cardiovascular practice. The prevalence of TAA is estimated to be 6 persons per 100,000 per year.[1] TAA are most often clinically silent and identified incidentally on an imaging examination. Initial symptoms of TAA are most often secondary to aortic dissection or rupture, potentially fatal conditions associated with TAA. In the United States, in 2018, just less than 10,000 deaths were attributed to aortic aneurysm, although this is likely an underestimate.[2,3] In this review, we provide a practical evidence-based summary of the pathophysiology, risk factors, associated genetic syndromes, and the clinical management of TAA.

PHYSIOLOGY AND PATHOPHYSIOLOGY
The Normal Aorta

The aorta is the primary conduit blood vessel supplying the systemic circulation of the human body. From the heart, the aorta courses through the thorax before descending below the diaphragm, delineating the thoracic from the abdominal aorta (**Fig. 1**). The thoracic aorta can be subdivided into 3 segments: the ascending aorta from the aortic valve to the take-off of the innominate artery, the aortic arch from the innominate artery origin to the origin of the left subclavian artery, and the descending aorta just past the left subclavian to the level of the diaphragm. Histologically, the aorta is composed of 3 distinct layers: a thin inner tunica intima, a thicker tunica media, and an outermost tunica adventitia. Normal aortic size varies based on age, sex, height, segment of aorta, imaging modality, and by imaging technique. In general, normal aortic diameter in adults should not exceed 40 mm.[4] Published reference values for the upper limit of normal of aortic diameter in adults eligible for low-dose computed tomography scan for lung cancer screening are sinotubular junction 4.08 (male [M])/3.83 (female [F]), midascending aorta 4.15 (M)/3.99 (F), transverse aorta 3.45 (M)/3.16 (F), mid-descending aorta 3.26 (M)/2.94 (F), and diaphragmatic hiatus 3.16 (M)/2.90 (F); with

[a] Heart and Vascular Center, Dartmouth-Hitchcock Medical Center, 1 Medical Center Drive, Lebanon, NH 03756, USA; [b] Department of Medicine, Dartmouth-Hitchcock Medical Center, 1 Medical Center Drive, Lebanon, NH 03756, USA
* Corresponding author.
E-mail address: Stanislav.henkin@hitchcock.org

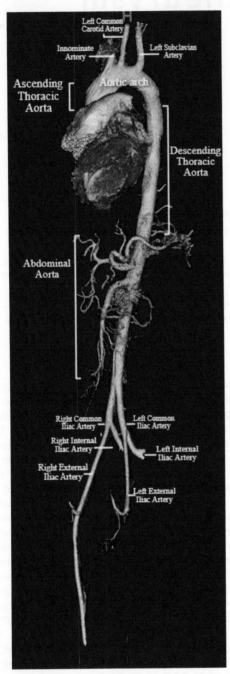

Fig. 1. Normal aortic anatomy.

all measurements in cm.[5] The rate of normal aortic expansion is approximately 0.9 mm and 0.7 mm per decade of life for men and women, respectively.[4]

DEFINITION OF THORACIC AORTIC ANEURYSMS

Strictly, a TAA must involve all 3 layers of the arterial wall and have at least a 50% increase in diameter when compared with the contiguous diameter.[6] Although this definition is widely accepted, it lacks an outcomes correlate. Additionally, many cases of aortic dilation severe enough to meet guideline recommendations for prophylactic repair, do not meet this strict definition.[7]

A TAA can be further defined by its location, morphology, and degree of aortic involvement. The majority of TAA involve the aortic root or ascending aorta (60%), whereas 40% involve the descending aorta, 10% involve the aortic arch, and 10% involve the thoracoabdominal aorta.[8] TAA most often have a fusiform morphology, characterized by symmetric dilation that is pancircumferential. Less common, saccular aneurysms are localized outpouchings of the aortic wall and are more commonly associated with aortic infection, trauma, degeneration of an atherosclerotic ulcer, or a prior aortic surgery.[9]

PATHOPHYSIOLOGY, ETIOLOGY, AND NATURAL HISTORY OF THORACIC AORTIC ANEURYSMS

Aneurysms of the thoracic aorta arise by a process known as cystic medial necrosis or medial degeneration, characterized by a decrease in smooth muscle cells, break down of elastin fibers, and increased deposition of proteoglycans in the tunica media of the aortic wall.[1] As the aorta dilates, per Laplace's law, aortic wall stress increases proportionally. Ultimately, as medial degeneration progresses and aortic diameter increases, the risk of aortic complications increases.

The initial aneurysm size at time of diagnosis is the best predictor of growth rate and risk of rupture.[10] Studies on the natural history of TAA demonstrate a sharp acceleration or hinge point for the risk of rupture and dissection as the maximum aortic diameter exceeds 5.5 cm.[11–14] The risk of death, rupture, or dissection is 6.5% per year for TAA greater than 5 cm, and 14.1% per year for TAAs greater than 6.0 cm.[12] The average growth rate of TAA greatly exceeds that of normal aorta, averaging 0.10 cm per year (0.07 for ascending and 0.19 for descending).[12] The natural history of TAA also depends on the underlying etiology and genetics (**Fig. 2**).[15,16]

The majority of TAA are degenerative, occurring in association with long-standing increases in wall stress and traditional risk factors for atherosclerosis, including age, hypertension, hyperlipidemia, and smoking.[17,18] TAA of the descending aorta are often associated with atherosclerosis. A proportion of TAA (approximately 5%), particularly in the ascending aorta, are associated with inherited

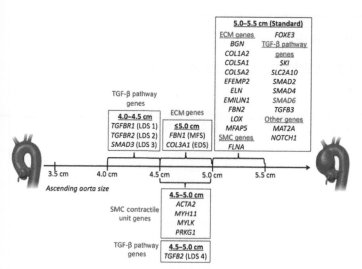

5.0–5.5 cm (Standard)	
ECM genes	FOXE3
BGN	TGF-β pathway
COL1A2	genes
COL5A1	SKI
COL5A2	SLC2A10
EFEMP2	SMAD2
ELN	SMAD4
EMILIN1	SMAD6
FBN2	TGFB3
LOX	Other genes
MFAP5	MAT2A
	NOTCH1

TGF-β pathway genes

4.0–4.5 cm
TGFBR1 (LDS 1)
TGFBR2 (LDS 2)
SMAD3 (LDS 3)

ECM genes
≤5.0 cm
FBN1 (MFS)
COL3A1 (EDS)

SMC genes
FLNA

3.5 cm   4.0 cm   4.5 cm   5.0 cm   5.5 cm

Ascending aorta size

4.5–5.0 cm
ACTA2
MYH11
MYLK
PRKG1

SMC contractile unit genes

TGF-β pathway genes

4.5–5.0 cm
TGFB2 (LDS 4)

Fig. 2. Genetics and aortic diameter determines threshold for ascending TAA repair. (From Brownstein AJ, Kostiuk V, Ziganshin BA, et al. Genes Associated with Thoracic Aortic Aneurysm and Dissection: 2018 Update and Clinical Implications. Aorta (Stamford). 2018;6(1):13 to 20; with permission.)

disorders of connective tissue, bicuspid aortic valves (**Fig. 3**), and familial/genetic predisposition (**Table 1**). Although less common, healed aortic dissection, aortic coarctation, and aortitis are also important etiologies of TAA. Aortitis can be secondary to autoimmune diseases (giant cell arteritis, Takayasu arteritis, Behçet's disease, seronegative spondyloarthropathies, or IgG4 related) or infectious diseases (syphilis, mycotic aneurysms from staphylococcus or salmonella, and tuberculosis).

More than 20% of patients with TAA or dissection report a family history of TAA, supporting a strong genetic predisposition for the disease, most often inherited in an autosomal dominant pattern.[11,19] Familial TAA do not have systemic clinical features that characterize inherited connective tissue disorders. Patients with TAA in the setting of Marfan syndrome (MFS), Loeys–Dietz syndrome (LDS), vascular Ehlers–Danlos syndrome, or familial TAA have abnormally high risk for aortic dissection and rupture, even at a younger age and relatively modest aortic diameters.[20,21]

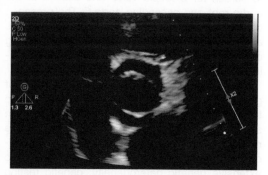

Fig. 3. A transthoracic echocardiogram, parasternal short axis, demonstrating a bicuspid aortic valve.

- Initial aneurysm size at time of diagnosis is the best predictor of growth rate and risk of rupture.[10]
- The natural history of TAA also depends on the underlying etiology and genetics.[15,16]
- Patients with TAA with MFS, LDS, vascular Ehlers–Danlos syndrome, or familial TAA have an abnormally high risk for aortic dissection and rupture, even at a younger age and relatively modest aortic diameters.

CLINICAL PRESENTATION OF THORACIC AORTIC ANEURYSMS

More than 95% of TAA are asymptomatic until the point of dissection or rupture.[22] Regardless of diameter, the development of symptoms attributed to TAA should prompt an urgent evaluation for surgical repair.[6] A variety of symptom complexes can result, depending on the size and position of the TAA. Clinical heart failure and a diastolic murmur can occur in the setting of severe aortic regurgitation secondary to aneurysm of the aortic root. Chest pain may develop secondary to compression of surrounding structures and erosion into adjacent bones. Aneurysm of the aortic arch and descending aorta can both rarely compress the mainstem bronchus or esophagus causing dyspnea or dysphagia, respectively. Descending aortic aneurysms can cause back pain and erode into the thoracic vertebral bodies.

TAA rupture most often presents as acute severe chest pain, hypotension, and hemorrhagic shock. Less commonly, rupture can occur into the esophagus causing hematemesis; in the bronchus causing massive hemoptysis; or through a sinus of Valsalva resulting in aortic fistula into the

Table 1
Genetic syndromes associated with TAA and dissection

Genetic Syndrome	Genetic Defect(s)	Common Clinical Features
MFS	FBN1	Ectopia lentis Dural ectasia Overgrowth of long bones
Loyes–Dietz syndrome	TGFBR1 or TGFBR2	Bifid uvula or cleft palate Arterial tortuosity Hypertelorism Craniosynostosis Skeletal features similar to MFS Aneurysms/dissections of other arteries
Vascular Ehlers–Danlos	COL3A1	Thin, translucent skin Gastrointestinal rupture Rupture of the gravid uterus Rupture of medium and large arteries
Turner syndrome	45, X karyotype	Short stature Primary amenorrhea Bicuspid aortic valve Aortic coarctation Webbed neck, lock set ears, low hairline, broad chest
Familial TAA and dissection[a]	TGFBR2	Thin translucent skin Arterial or aortic tortuosity Arterial aneurysms
	MYH11 ACTA2	Patent ductus arteriosus Livedo reticularis Iris flocculi Patent ductus arteriosus Bicuspid aortic valve
	MYLK	

Abbreviations: ACTA2, actin, alpha 2, smooth muscle aorta; COL3A1, type III collagen; FBN1, fibrillin 1; MFS, Marfan syndrome; MYH 11, smooth muscle specific beta-myosin heavy chain; MYLK, myosin light chain kinase; TGFBR1, transforming growth factor-beta receptor type I; TGFBR2, transforming growth factor-beta receptor type II.

[a] Increasing number of definite mutations and mutations of variable associated risk have been identified.[16]

(Adapted from Tables 6 and 7 from Hiratzka LF, Bakris GL, Beckman JA, et al. 2010 ACCF/AHA/AATS/ACR/ASA/SCA/SCAI/SIR/STS/SVM guidelines for the diagnosis and management of patients with thoracic aortic disease, with permission from the American Heart Association.)

right atrium, right ventricle, or pulmonary artery with subsequent heart failure.

- More than 95% of TAA are asymptomatic until the point of dissection or rupture.[22]

SCREENING

The diagnosis of TAA is most frequently made incidentally, and to a lesser extent by screening.[4] Unlike for abdominal aortic aneurysm, there is no TAA screening recommendation for the general population. However, guidelines recommend screening first-degree relatives of patients with a history TAA or aortic dissection.[4,6,23,24] If there is extensive evidence of a familial TAA, then screening second-degree relatives is reasonable.[6,23] Screening for TAA may also be reasonable in patients with first-degree relatives with unexplained sudden cardiac death.[6,23]

In first-degree relatives of patients with bicuspid aortic valve, an echocardiogram is recommended to screen for bicuspid valve and dilation of the aortic root and ascending aorta.[25] The presence of aneurysm at other anatomic locations, such as an intracranial aneurysm, may warrant full imaging of the aorta owing to a relatively high rate of coexistent sites of pathology.[26]

Screening is accomplished by a combination of genetic testing and aortic imaging. Upfront genetic testing of the proband with next-generation sequencing, with cascade testing of first-degree relatives if a mutation is discovered, is both efficient and cost effective.[15] However, owing to extensive genetic heterogeneity, genetic testing may not consistently yield a pathologic mutation despite the high likelihood of genetic transmission.[11,23] Thus, even with negative genetic testing, a screening imaging test may be indicated if clinical suspicious remains high.[6,24]

Owing to the high prevalence of aneurysms at other sites beyond the thoracic aorta in patients with familial TAA, computed tomography angiography (CTA) or magnetic resonance angiography (MRA) should be obtained to image the entire aorta. A transthoracic echocardiogram (TTE) should be obtained to screen for valvular disease. Screening with imaging is reasonable by age 25 or 10 years before the youngest case in a family cluster.[6,24] If initial screening is normal, reimaging should occur at 5-year intervals.[23] If serial imaging is expected to continue, MRA may be preferred over CTA to avoid ionizing radiation.[6]

- Guidelines recommend screening of first-degree relatives of patients with a history of TAA or aortic dissection and screening second-degree relatives if there is extensive evidence of a familial TAA and dissection.

IMAGING

The ability to completely and accurately image the aorta is essential for the diagnosis, screening, surveillance, and management of TAA. Therefore, clinicians caring for patients with TAA should have an understanding of the basic principles of aortic imaging. This should include an awareness of recommendations for screening and surveillance, in addition to the strengths and weakness of the available imaging modalities.

Surveillance

Periodic imaging of TAA should be performed to determine the necessity and timing of prophylactic surgery.[4,6,7,24] Surveillance imaging of TAA should ensure accurate measurement of the maximal aortic diameter, while minimizing costs, time burden, and potential harm to patients.

The rate of aneurysm growth has been associated with an increased need for prophylactic surgery and risk dissection or rupture.[18] A rapid TAA growth rate (>0.5 cm in 6 months or >1 cm in 1 year) can be the sole indication or modifying factor for proceeding with prophylactic repair.[4,6,27] When comparing serial imaging, it is important to ensure comparisons are made at the same location, using the same technique of measurement, with the same modality of imaging when reporting TAA growth rate. Measurements in aortic wall thickness can vary by 0.2 to 0.4 cm depending on whether echocardiography, CTA, or MRA is used.[28] An understanding of the strengths and

weaknesses of the different imaging modalities are key when selecting and interpreting imaging in patients with TAA (**Table 2**).

The 2015 guidelines from the American Society of Echocardiography and European Society of Cardiac Imaging offer detailed recommendations for surveillance of TAA. In general, newly discovered TAA or those nearing threshold for surgical intervention should be reimaged in 6 months to establish stability. TTE can be used for serial imaging of the dilated aortic root and proximal ascending aorta, but only when there is established agreement between measurements on TTE and CTA or MRA.[7] TAAs that are stable in size can be imaged annually or every 2 to 3 years depending on individualized risk. In patients with MFS, biannual imaging is recommended unless the TAA is stable, less than 4.5 cm, and the patient has no family history of dissection.[7] In lower risk patients with MFS, repeat CTA or MRA is suggested every 2 to 3 years to reassess the aortic arch and descending aorta.[4,7]

- Newly discovered TAA or those nearing threshold for surgical intervention should be reimaged in 6 months, and TAA that are stable in size can be imaged annually or every 2 to 3 years depending on individualized risk.

Imaging Techniques

When weighing possible surgical referral, whether based on aortic diameter or growth rate, it is of paramount importance that measurements are accurate and consistent. Common pitfalls that can result in flawed measurements include oblique measurements, overmeasurement of the anterior aortic wall on TTE, and comparing diameters from studies that used different measuring techniques. Ensuring adherence to guideline recommendations for aortic imaging and measurement is essential to avoid these types of errors in clinical practice. Reviewing imaging independently or with a thoracic radiologist can decrease errors.

For all imaging modalities, it is recommended to measure the aortic diameter perpendicular to the axis of blood flow or perpendicular to the longitudinal axis of the aorta.[7] Oblique measurements lead to inflation of the reported aortic diameter and consequent inappropriate surgical referral.

Measurement by TTE should be performed in end-diastole from the leading edge of the anterior aortic wall to the leading edge of the posterior aortic wall (**Fig. 4**).[29] Most studies on the natural history of TAA of the aortic root and ascending aorta have used TTE for measurements.[11–13,30]

Unfortunately, there is no standard recommendation for how to measure aortic diameter by

Table 2
Most common imaging modalities used for diagnosis and surveillance of TAA with associated advantages and disadvantages

Modality	Advantages	Disadvantages
CTA	Visualizes all aortic segments and branch vessels. Accurate and reproducible. Best spatial resolution. Quick and widely available. Less expensive than MRI. Preferred for patients with prior aortic surgery.	Ionizing radiation. Incidental findings. Requires iodinated contrast.
MRA	Visualizes all aortic segments and branch vessels. Accurate and reproducible. Best at visualizing pathology of vessel wall, such as inflammation. No ionizing radiation	Most expensive and time consuming. Patient cooperation issues – breath-holding and/or claustrophobia. Magnetic susceptibility artifact from metallic material if prior graft or implant.
TTE	Quick and relatively cheap. No ionizing radiation. Usually diagnostic for aneurysms that effect the aortic root. Allows assessment of cardiac function and valvular disease.	Variable and incomplete visualization of the aorta risks missing the most severely dilated segment.

Abbreviations: CTA, computed tomography angiography; MRA, magnetic resonance angiography; TTE, transthoracic echocardiography.

CTA or MRA and variability exists in clinical practice. A 2016 study comparing measurements of the ascending aorta and aortic root by TTE and multidetector CT scans found that the diameters are consistently larger with multidetector CT scans; using a leading edge to leading edge method in both modalities resulted in the best correlation.[31] Despite this issue, CTA and MRA have many advantages over TTE, especially a complete visualization of the aorta and the ability to use 3-dimensional reconstructed images to prevent oblique measurement (**Fig. 5**).

Indexing Measurements

Almost 60% of patients with type A aortic dissection present at a diameter less than 5.5 cm, which are smaller than the current recommendations for prophylactic repair.[32] There is some evidence that indexed measurements of aortic diameter by body surface area or height improves risk stratification compared with unindexed measurements.[33] Indexing measurements is well-established for Turner syndrome and the pediatric MFS population, but is not widely adopted in adult clinical practice.

Aortic size indexed by height has been shown to correlate well with the risk of aortic dissection (**Fig. 6**), and could be of use particularly in patients at the lower and upper extremes of stature.[33]

MEDICAL THERAPY AND RISK FACTOR MANAGEMENT

Medical therapy and risk factor modification are important tools to slow the rate of growth of TAA and may be the only option for individuals deemed too high risk for surgical intervention. Despite only moderate to poor quality evidence, optimal treatment of hypertension, hyperlipidemia, and coexisting atherosclerotic disease are class I recommendations for all patients with TAA.[6,24] Smoking cessation is of vast importance because the rate of thoracic aneurysm expansion is nearly doubled in active smokers.[18]

Beta blockers have been shown to slow the rate of TAA expansion in patients with MFS, but not in degenerative TAA, limiting generalizability.[34–37] Current guidelines recommend treatment of all patients with MFS with a beta blocker to reduce the

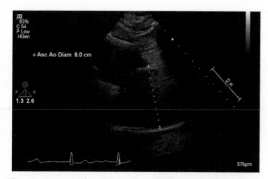

Fig. 4. A transthoracic echocardiogram, parasternal long axis, showing a 6-cm ascending aortic aneurysm. Note the measurement is performed in end-diastole, leading edge to leading edge.

rate of aortic dilation.[4,6,24] Despite the narrow indication, beta blockers are widely prescribed in patients TAA without MFS.[17]

Angiotensin II receptor blockers (ARB) have more recently been discovered to decreased the progression of aortic dilation in patients with MFS. Several, mostly small, clinical studies have shown that ARB reduces the rate of growth of TAA in this population.[38–41] This finding has led to guideline recommendations for ARB use in all patients with MFS.[4,6,24] Additionally, there is strong evidence from preclinical models to suggest benefit for LDS.[42] However, much like beta blockers, there is little evidence to suggest ARB are efficacious for patients with TAA without MFS or LDS. The benefits of beta-blockers and ARB may attenuate with larger TAA.[6,36]

The optimal blood pressure target for patients with TAA remains unclear. Although clinicians may consider treating blood pressure more aggressively, large clinical trials of hypertension did not track aortic outcomes and there is no evidence to support lower blood pressure targets in TAA than those put forth in current hypertension guidelines.[43]

- The optimal treatment of hypertension, coexisting atherosclerotic disease, and smoking cessation are class I recommendations for all patients with TAA.
- Beta blockers and ARBs slow the growth of TAA in MFS, but benefit is not proven in the wider population with TAA.

WHEN TO INTERVENE

Prophylactic operative repair of large aortic aneurysms is the most effective means for the prevention of aortic rupture and aortic dissection. Patients discharged from the hospital after successful TAA repair have similar long-term mortality rates compared with age- and sex-matched controls.[33] Guideline recommendations for thresholds to consider prophylactic intervention are based on current understanding of the natural history of TAA and the risks associated with the operation (**Table 3**).[11] Regardless of diameter, worrisome symptoms like chest or back pain that may be related to TAA should prompt evaluation for surgical repair.[6]

Open repair remains the gold standard treatment of large TAA of the ascending aorta and the aortic arch. Elective open surgical repair of TAA carries a 3% risk of lasting morbidity (especially stroke) and 3% risk of mortality even at high volume centers.[44] This finding compares favorably to the 22% in hospital mortality rate for surgery for type A aortic dissection, which does not include patients who expire before surgery.[45] Patients who undergo open TAA repair in lower volume centers have increased risk of in-hospital mortality compared with those undergoing the operation at high volume centers.[46] Thus,

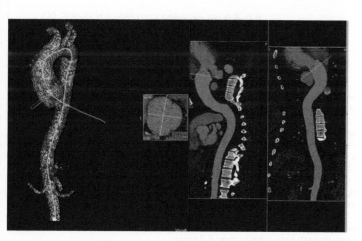

Fig. 5. Three-dimensional computed tomography angiography reconstruction of the aortic root and ascending aortic aneurysm.

		Aortic Size (cm)									
		3.5	4.0	4.5	5.0	5.5	6.0	6.5	7.0	7.5	8.0
Height (inches) (m)											
55	1.40	2.50	2.86	3.21	3.57	3.93	4.29	4.64	5.00	5.36	5.71
57	1.45	2.41	2.76	3.10	3.45	3.79	4.14	4.48	4.83	5.17	5.52
59	1.50	2.33	2.67	3.00	3.33	3.67	4.00	4.33	4.67	5.00	5.33
61	1.55	2.26	2.58	2.90	3.23	3.55	3.87	4.19	4.52	4.84	5.16
63	1.60	2.19	2.50	2.81	3.13	3.44	3.75	4.06	4.38	4.69	5.00
65	1.65	2.12	2.42	2.73	3.03	3.33	3.64	3.94	4.24	4.55	4.85
67	1.70	2.06	2.35	2.65	2.94	3.24	3.53	3.82	4.12	4.41	4.71
69	1.75	2.00	2.29	2.57	2.86	3.14	3.43	3.71	4.00	4.29	4.57
71	1.80	1.94	2.22	2.50	2.78	3.06	3.33	3.61	3.89	4.17	4.44
73	1.85	1.89	2.16	2.43	2.70	2.97	3.24	3.51	3.78	4.05	4.32
75	1.90	1.84	2.11	2.37	2.63	2.89	3.16	3.42	3.68	3.95	4.21
77	1.95	1.79	2.05	2.31	2.56	2.82	3.08	3.33	3.59	3.85	4.10
79	2.00	1.75	2.00	2.25	2.50	2.75	3.00	3.25	3.50	3.75	4.00
81	2.05	1.71	1.95	2.20	2.44	2.68	2.93	3.17	3.41	3.66	3.90

= low risk (~ 4% per year)   = moderate risk (~ 7% per year)   = High risk (~ 12% per year)   = severe risk (~ 18% per year)

Light green area indicates low risk, yellow area indicates moderate risk, orange area indicates high risk, and red area indicates severe risk.

Fig. 6. Nomogram of risk of aortic dissection by aortic diameter indexed to height. From Zafar MA, Li Y, Rizzo JA, et al. Height alone, rather than body surface area, suffices for risk estimation in ascending aortic aneurysm. J Thorac Cardiovasc Surg. 2018; with permission.

Table 3
Current guideline recommended thresholds for prophylactic repair of TAA

Condition	Threshold for Intervention
Degenerative TAA	
Aortic root or ascending aortic aneurysm	5.5 cm [ACC, CCS, ESC]
Aortic arch aneurysm	5.5 cm [ESC, ACC], 6.0 cm [CCS]
Descending aortic aneurysm	5.5 cm (TEVAR)[ACC, ESC], 6.0 cm [ACC, ESC] 6.5 cm [CCS]
Accelerated rate of growth	≥0.5 cm/y [ACC, CCS]
Undergoing cardiac surgery for other reasons	4.5 cm [ACC, CCS, ESC]
BAV	5.5 cm [ACCα, CCS, ESC] or $\pi r^2/H > 10$ [ACCα]
BAV + additional risk factors/low surgical risk[a]	5.0 cm [ACCα, CCS, ESC]
Genetic syndromes	
MFS	4.0–5.0 cm or $\pi r^2/H > 10$ [ACC]; 5.0 cm [ESC, CCS]
MFS + anticipated pregnancy	4.0 cm [ACC]; 4.5 cm [ESC]; 4.1–4.5 cm [CCS]
MFS + additional risk factors[b]	4.5 cm [ESC]
v-EDS or Turner syndrome	4.5–5.0 cm [CCS]
LDS	4.2 cm (TEE) or 4.4–4.6 cm (CTA/MRA) [ACC]
Familial TAA	4.5–5.0 cm [ACC, CCS], or $\pi r^2/H > 10$ [ACC]

[ACC] 2010 ACCF/AHA/AATS/ACR/ASA/SCA/SCAI/SIR/STS/SVM guidelines for the diagnosis and management of patients with thoracic aortic disease.
[ACCα] 2014 AHA/ACC guideline for the management of patients with valvular heart disease: a report of the American College of Cardiology/American Heart Association Task Force on Practice Guidelines.
[CCS] 2014 Canadian Cardiovascular Society Position Statement on the Management of Thoracic Aortic Disease.
[ESC] 2014 European Society of Cardiology Guidelines on the Diagnosis and Treatment of Aortic Diseases.
Abbreviations: BAV, bicuspid aortic valve; CTA, computed tomography angiography; FTAAD, familial thoracic aneurysm and dissection; H, patient height in meters; LDS, Loeys-Dietz Syndrome; MFS, Marfan syndrome; MRA, magnetic resonance angiography; TEE, transesophageal echocardiography; TEVAR, thoracic endovascular aortic repair; v-EDS, vascular Ehlers–Danlos syndrome.
[a] Family history of aortic dissection, growth rate ≥0.5 cm/y, or low surgical risk.
[b] Family history of thoracic aortic dissection, growth rate greater than 0.3 cm/y.

consideration of referral to a tertiary center with expertise in TAA repair is reasonable.

Thoracic endovascular aortic repair (TEVAR) is a minimally invasive technique that has largely replaced traditional open operations for TAA of the descending aorta.[44] TEVAR has lower morbidity and mortality rates than open repair.[44] TEVAR into the aortic arch or ascending aorta can be used in high-risk patients, but requires fenestrated grafts or consideration of concomitant bypass of the arch branch vessels.[47,48] In connective tissue diseases such as MFS, open repair is preferred over TEVAR owing to a high risk of early and midterm complications and reinterventions.[49]

- Prophylactic operative repair of large aortic aneurysms is the most effective means for prevention of aortic rupture and aortic dissection.
- Open surgical repair is the gold standard for TAA of the ascending aorta and aortic arch, but TEVAR is now preferred for TAA of the descending aorta in the absence of inherited connective tissue disease.

SUMMARY

TAA is a common clinical entity with the potential for sudden catastrophic complications in the form of acute aortic dissection or aortic rupture. Inherited disorders of connective tissue and certain genetic mutations are associated with a more malignant natural history of TAA and should be managed more aggressively. Diagnosis and subsequent surveillance imaging is necessary to decrease the rates of aortic complications, primarily by means of referral for prophylactic aortic surgery.

CLINICS CARE POINTS

- Guidelines recommend screening for thoracic aortic aneurysm in first degree relatives of patients with a history of TAA or aortic dissection. Screening is also recommended in second degree relatives if there is extensive evidence of a familial predisposition.

- Newly discovered thoracic aortic aneurysms or those nearing the threshold for surgical intervention should be re-imaged in 6 months. TAA that are stable in size can be imaged annually or every 2-3 years depending on individualized risk.

- Optimal treatment of hypertension, coexisting atherosclerotic disease, and smoking cessation are class I recommendations for all patients with thoracic aortic aneurysm.

- Beta blockers and angiotensin receptor blockers slow the growth of thoracic aortic aneurysm in patients with Marfan Syndrome, but benefits are unproven in the wider population with TAA.

- Prophylactic operative repair of large TAA is the most effective means of prevention of aortic rupture and aortic dissection.

DISCLOSURE

The authors have nothing to disclose.

REFERENCES

1. Ince H, Nienaber CA. Etiology, pathogenesis and management of thoracic aortic aneurysm. Nat Clin Pract Cardiovasc Med 2007;4(8):418–27.
2. Centers for Disease Control and Prevention, National Center for Health Statistics. Underlying cause of death 1999–2018. Available at: http://wonder.cdc.gov/ucd-icd10.html. Accessed January 5, 2021.
3. Tanaka Y, Sakata K, Sakurai Y, et al. Prevalence of type A acute aortic dissection in patients with out-of-hospital cardiopulmonary arrest. Am J Cardiol 2016;117(11):1826–30.
4. Erbel R, Aboyans V, Boileau C, et al. 2014 ESC guidelines on the diagnosis and treatment of aortic diseases. Eur Heart J 2014;35(41):2873–926.
5. McComb BL, Munden RF, Duan F, et al. Normative reference values of thoracic aortic diameter in American College of Radiology imaging Network (ACRIN 6654) arm of National Lung Screening trial. Clin Imaging 2016;40(5):936–43.
6. Hiratzka LF, Bakris GL, Beckman JA, et al. 2010 ACCF/AHA/AATS/ACR/ASA/SCA/SCAI/SIR/STS/SVM guidelines for the diagnosis and management of patients with thoracic aortic disease. Circulation 2010;121(13). https://doi.org/10.1161/CIR.0b013e3181d4739e.
7. Goldstein SA, Evangelista A, Abbara S, et al. Multimodality imaging of diseases of the thoracic aorta in adults. J Am Soc Echocardiogr 2015;28(2):119–82.
8. Isselbacher EM. Thoracic and abdominal aortic aneurysms. Circulation 2005;111(6). https://doi.org/10.1161/01.CIR.0000154569.08857.7A.
9. Shang EK, Nathan DP, Boonn WW, et al. A modern experience with saccular aortic aneurysms. J Vasc Surg 2013;57(1):84–8.
10. Kim JB, Kim K, Lindsay ME, et al. Risk of rupture or dissection in descending thoracic aortic aneurysm. Circulation 2015;132:1620–9.

11. Coady MA, Rizzo JA, Hammond GL, et al. Surgical intervention criteria for thoracic aortic aneurysms: a study of growth rates and complications. Ann Thorac Surg 1999;67(6). https://doi.org/10.1016/S0003-4975(99)00431-2.

12. Elefteriades JA. Natural history of thoracic aortic aneurysms: indications for surgery, and surgical versus nonsurgical risks. Ann Thorac Surg 2002; 74(5). https://doi.org/10.1016/S0003-4975(02)04147-4.

13. Coady MA, Rizzo JA, Hammond GL, et al. What is the appropriate size criterion for resection of thoracic aortic aneurysms? J Thorac Cardiovasc Surg 1997;113(3). https://doi.org/10.1016/S0022-5223(97)70360-X.

14. Kouchoukos NT, Dougenis D. Surgery of the thoracic aorta. N Engl J Med 1997;336(26). https://doi.org/10.1056/NEJM199706263362606.

15. Brownstein AJ, Kostiuk V, Ziganshin BA, et al. Genes associated with thoracic aortic aneurysm and dissection: 2018 update and clinical implications. Aorta (Stamford) 2018;6(1):13–20.

16. Pinard A, Jones GT, Milewicz DM. Genetics of thoracic and abdominal aortic diseases. Circ Res 2019;124(4):588–606.

17. Braverman AC. Acute aortic dissection: clinician update. Circulation 2010;122(2):184–8.

18. Dapunt OE, Galla JD, Sadeghi AM, et al. The natural history of thoracic aortic aneurysms. J Thorac Cardiovasc Surg 1994;107(5):1323–33.

19. Albornoz G, Coady MA, Roberts M, et al. Familial thoracic aortic aneurysms and dissections-Incidence, modes of inheritance, and phenotypic patterns. Ann Thorac Surg 2006;82(4):1400–5.

20. Gott VL, Greene PS, Alejo DE, et al. Replacement of the aortic root in patients with Marfan's syndrome. N Engl J Med 1999;340(17). https://doi.org/10.1056/NEJM199904293401702.

21. Loeys BL, Schwarze U, Holm T, et al. Aneurysm syndromes caused by mutations in the TGF-β receptor. N Engl J Med 2006;355(8). https://doi.org/10.1056/NEJMoa055695.

22. Kuzmik GA, Sang AX, Elefteriades JA. Natural history of thoracic aortic aneurysms. J Vasc Surg 2012;56(2). https://doi.org/10.1016/j.jvs.2012.04.053.

23. Verhagen JMA, Kempers M, Cozijnsen L, et al. Expert consensus recommendations on the cardiogenetic care for patients with thoracic aortic disease and their first-degree relatives. Int J Cardiol 2018; 258:243–8.

24. Boodhwani M, Andelfinger G, Leipsic J, et al. Canadian cardiovascular society position statement on the management of thoracic aortic disease. Can J Cardiol 2014;30(6):577–89.

25. Otto CM, Nishimura RA, Bonow RO, et al. 2020 ACC/AHA guideline for the management of patients with valvular heart disease: executive summary: a report of the American College of Cardiology/American Heart Association Joint Committee on clinical practice guidelines. Circulation 2021;143(5):e35–71.

26. Laukka D, Pan E, Fordell T, et al. Prevalence of thoracic aortic aneurysms and dilatations in patients with intracranial aneurysms. J Vasc Surg 2019;70(6). https://doi.org/10.1016/j.jvs.2019.01.066.

27. 2010 ACCF/AHA/AATS/ACR/ASA/SCA/SCAI/SIR/STS/SVM GUIDELINES FOR THE DIAGNOSIS AND MANAGEMENT OF PATIENTS WITH THORACIC AORTIC DISEASE REPRESENTATIVE MEMBERS*, Hiratzka LF, Creager MA, Isselbacher EM, Svensson LG, 2014 AHA/ACC Guideline for the Management of Patients With Valvular Heart Disease Representative Members*, Nishimura RA, Bonow RO, Guyton RA, Sundt TM 3rd, ACC/AHA TASK FORCE MEMBERS, Halperin JL, Levine GN, Anderson JL, Albert NM, Al-Khatib SM, Birtcher KK, Bozkurt B, Brindis RG, Cigarroa JE, Curtis LH, Fleisher LA, Gentile F, Gidding S, Hlatky MA, Ikonomidis J, Joglar J, Kovacs RJ, Ohman EM, Pressler SJ, Sellke FW, Shen WK, Wijeysundera DN. Surgery for aortic dilatation in patients with bicuspid aortic valves: a statement of clarification from the American College of Cardiology/American heart association Task Force on clinical practice guidelines. Circulation 2016;133(7): 680–6.

28. Goldfinger JZ, Halperin JL, Marin ML, et al. Thoracic aortic aneurysm and dissection. J Am Coll Cardiol 2014;64(16). https://doi.org/10.1016/j.jacc.2014.08.025.

29. Sahn DJ, DeMaria A, Kisslo J, et al. Recommendations regarding quantitation in M-mode echocardiography: results of a survey of echocardiographic measurements. Circulation 1978;58(6). https://doi.org/10.1161/01.CIR.58.6.1072.

30. Davies RR, Goldstein LJ, Coady MA, et al. Yearly rupture or dissection rates for thoracic aortic aneurysms: simple prediction based on size. Ann Thorac Surg 2002;73(1). https://doi.org/10.1016/S0003-4975(01)03236-2.

31. Blondheim DS, Vassilenko L, Glick Y, et al. Aortic dimensions by multi-detector computed tomography vs. echocardiography. J Cardiol 2016;67(4):365–70.

32. Pape LA, Tsai TT, Isselbacher EM, et al. Aortic diameter ≥5.5 cm is not a good predictor of type A aortic dissection: observations from the International Registry of Acute Aortic Dissection (IRAD). Circulation 2007;116(10):1120–7.

33. Zafar MA, Li Y, Rizzo JA, et al. Height alone, rather than body surface area, suffices for risk estimation in ascending aortic aneurysm. J Thorac Cardiovasc Surg 2018;155(5):1938–50.

34. Silverman DI, Burton KJ, Gray J, et al. Life expectancy in the Marfan syndrome. Am J Cardiol 1995;

75(2). https://doi.org/10.1016/S0002-9149(00)80066-1.

35. Salim MA, Alpert BS, Ward JC, et al. Effect of beta-adrenergic blockade on aortic root rate of dilation in the Marfan syndrome. Am J Cardiol 1994;74(6). https://doi.org/10.1016/0002-9149(94)90762-5.

36. Shores J, Berger KR, Murphy EA, et al. Progression of aortic dilatation and the benefit of long-term β-adrenergic blockade in Marfan's syndrome. N Engl J Med 1994;330(19). https://doi.org/10.1056/NEJM199405123301902.

37. Ladouceur M, Fermanian C, Lupoglazoff JM, et al. Effect of beta-blockade on ascending aortic dilatation in children with the Marfan syndrome. Am J Cardiol 2007;99(3):406–9.

38. Groenink M, den Hartog AW, Franken R, et al. Losartan reduces aortic dilatation rate in adults with Marfan syndrome: a randomized controlled trial. Eur Heart J 2013;34(45). https://doi.org/10.1093/eurheartj/eht334.

39. Pees C, Laccone F, Hagl M, et al. Usefulness of losartan on the size of the ascending aorta in an unselected cohort of children, adolescents, and young adults with Marfan syndrome. Am J Cardiol 2013;112(9). https://doi.org/10.1016/j.amjcard.2013.06.019.

40. Brooke BS, Habashi JP, Judge DP, et al. Angiotensin II blockade and aortic-root dilation in Marfan's syndrome. N Engl J Med 2008;358(26). https://doi.org/10.1056/NEJMoa0706585.

41. Mullen M, Jin XY, Child A, et al. AIMS Investigators. Irbesartan in Marfan syndrome (AIMS): a double-blind, placebo-controlled randomised trial. Lancet 2019;394(10216):2263–70.

42. Gallo EM, Loch DC, Habashi JP, et al. Angiotensin II-dependent TGF-β signaling contributes to Loeys-Dietz syndrome vascular pathogenesis. J Clin Invest 2014;124(1):448–60.

43. Unger T, Borghi C, Charchar F, et al. 2020 International society of hypertension global hypertension practice guidelines. Hypertension 2020;75(6). https://doi.org/10.1161/HYPERTENSIONAHA.120.15026.

44. Tan G, Khoo P, Chan K. A review of endovascular treatment of thoracic aorta disease [published online ahead of print, 2018 Oct 5]. Ann R Coll Surg Engl 2018;100(8):1–6.

45. Evangelista A, Isselbacher EM, Bossone E, et al. Insights from the international registry of acute aortic dissection: a 20-year experience of collaborative clinical research. Circulation 2018;137(17):1846–60.

46. Nam K, Jang EJ, Jo JW, et al. Association between institutional case volume and mortality following thoracic aorta replacement: a nationwide Korean cohort study. J Cardiothorac Surg 2020;15(1):156.

47. Nation DA, Wang GJ. TEVAR: endovascular repair of the thoracic aorta. Semin Intervent Radiol 2015;32(3):265–71.

48. Zhu J, Dai X, Noiniyom P, et al. Fenestrated thoracic endovascular aortic repair using physician-modified stent grafts (PMSGs) in Zone 0 and Zone 1 for aortic arch diseases. Cardiovasc Intervent Radiol 2019;42(1):19–27.

49. Gagné-Loranger M, Voisine P, Dagenais F. Should endovascular therapy Be considered for patients with connective tissue disorder? Can J Cardiol 2016;32(1):1–3.

Abdominal Aortic and Visceral Artery Aneurysms

Indrani Sen, MD[a], Camila Franco-Mesa, MD[b], Young Erben, MD[b],
Randall R. DeMartino, MD, MS[a,*]

KEYWORDS

- Aortic aneurysm • Visceral aneurysm • Epidemiology • Endovascular

KEY POINTS

- Abdominal aortic aneurysms are most common in men, and associated with increased age and a history of smoking.
- Screening can decrease abdominal aortic aneurysm–related mortality.
- Elective abdominal aortic aneurysm repair is considered at a size of greater than 5.5 cm, presence of symptoms, rapid expansion, or saccular morphology, and can be accomplished by open or endovascular approaches.
- Visceral artery aneurysms of the hepatic, splenic, and mesenteric circulation are often found incidentally.
- Visceral artery aneurysms should be repaired when they exceed 2 to 3 cm, are symptomatic, found in pregnancy or women of childbearing age, or are pseudoaneurysms.

ABDOMINAL AORTIC ANEURYSMS
Epidemiology and Incidence

Abdominal aortic aneurysm (AAA) is defined as a maximal diameter of the abdominal aorta of more than 3 cm, or a focal abnormal dilatation of the abdominal aorta greater than 1.5 times the normal adjacent arterial segment.[1,2] Although this is a generalized definition, normal aortic size is known to vary with sex, ethnicity, and age, with the aorta becoming aneurysmal at the smaller absolute size in women.[2] Multisite aortic aneurysms occur in 3% to 10% of patients, with the descending thoracic aorta and the infrarenal aorta being the most frequent sites of concurrent involvement.[3] Involvement of the suprarenal aorta is present in 5% to 15% of patients. The estimated prevalence of AAA from historical population-based studies varies from 2% to 18% in males and 0% to 4%

in females, with autopsy studies reporting a frequency of 0.5% to 3.0%. Mortality associated with AAA stems from its natural history of growth with subsequent rupture.[4–6] Only one-half the patients with rupture survive to reach the hospital, and most do not have an antecedent diagnosis of AAA. In those with ruptured AAA, the traditional treatment option was emergency open repair with a high (50%) intraoperative mortality, as compared with a mortality rate of 1% with elective repair. Worldwide, multiple studies have demonstrated the benefit of ultrasound-based screening for the identification of aneurysms with a decrease in aneurysm-related and all-cause mortality. These studies included the Chichester and The Multicentre Aneurysm Screening Study (MASS) (UK), Viborg (Denmark), Western Australia, Veteran's (United States), Rotterdam (the Netherlands), and Tromso (Norway) studies (**Table 1**).[7–12]

Physical address: Division of Vascular and Endovascular Surgery – Gonda Vascular Center – Mayo Clinic 200 First Street SW, 55905 – Rochester MN (USA).

Conflict of interests: None.

Funding: none.

[a] Division of Vascular and Endovascular Surgery, Mayo Clinic, 200 2nd Street SW, Rochester, MN 55902, USA;
[b] Department of Vascular Surgery, Mayo Clinic, 4500 San Pablo Road, Jacksonville, FL 32224, USA
* Corresponding author.
E-mail address: DeMartino.Randall@mayo.edu

Cardiol Clin 39 (2021) 517–525
https://doi.org/10.1016/j.ccl.2021.06.004

Table 1
Results of screening studies[15,54,55,56]

Study, Country, year	Prevalence of AAA	Follow-up Duration	Mortality*
Chichester, UK, 1995	4.0% (7.6% men, 1.3% women)	2.5 y	0.59 (0.27–1.29)
Rotterdam, the Netherlands, 1995	4.1% men, 0.7% women	—	
Tromso, Norway, 2001	8.9% men, 2.2% women	—	6% (all cause) at 120 mo
Viborg, Denmark, 2002	4.0%	5.1 y	0.31 (0.13–0.79)
MASS UK, 2002	4.9%	4.1 y	0.58 (0.42–0.78)
Western Australia, 2004	7.2%	3.6 y	0.72 (0.39–1.32)

* Aortic-related mortality at last follow-up, hazard or risk ratio, screened versus not, 95% confidence interval (CI); pooled odds ratio (OR) showed a decrease in AAA-related mortality favoring screening (OR, 0.57 [95% CI, 0.45–0.74]).

Introduction of population surveillance programs, measures to decrease smoking, and the introduction of endovascular therapy has dramatically decreased the incidence and mortality of AAA.[13] The estimated annual risk of abdominal aortic rupture is closely correlated with maximal aortic diameter as presented in **Table 2**.[14]

Risk Factors

The common etiology for AAAs is degenerative, which is associated with atherosclerosis. The major risk factors associated with AAAs are history of smoking, older age, male sex, Caucasian race, family history of AAA, hypertension, hypercholesterolemia, height, body mass index, chronic obstructive pulmonary disease, and atherosclerosis in other vascular territories (peripheral or coronary).[15] However, many of these factors are also markers for atherosclerosis burden and not specific risk factors for degenerative aneurysms. Smoking and tobacco use are most strongly associated with AAA, with the risk increasing significantly with the number of years of smoking.

Table 2
Rupture risk of AAAs (SVS guidelines, 2018)

Aneurysm size(cm)	Rupture Risk (%)
<4	0
4.0–4.9	0.5–5.0
5.0–5.9	3–15
6.0–6.9	10–20
7.0–7.9	20–40
>8	30–50

Data from Chaikof EL, Dalman RL, Eskandari MK, et al. The Society for Vascular Surgery practice guidelines on the care of patients with an abdominal aortic aneurysm. J Vasc Surg 2018;67(1):2-77.e72.

Smoking is also associated with continued aneurysm growth, and with reintervention after the initial treatment. The overall incidence of AAA in men is 4 to 6 times higher than in women, with disease onset up to a decade later in women. However, some of these differences decrease when aortic size is stratified by sex, age, and body surface area in women.[16] A positive family history of AAA, presence of aneurysms in other large vessels, and syndromic genetic disorders like Marfan syndrome, Ehlers–Danlos syndrome, and Loeys–Dietz syndrome are additional risk factors for AAA.

Screening and Surveillance

Aneurysms are usually asymptomatic. However, a pulsatile abdominal mass may be detected on clinical examination. Yet, the accuracy of clinical examination alone is poor in obese patients or in those with a small AAA. Ultrasound examination is safe and inexpensive and has high sensitivity (95%–100%) and specificity (100%) for detection of AAA. The Society for Vascular Surgery (SVS) recommends a one-time ultrasound screening for all men or women 65 to 75 years of age with a history of tobacco use (Grade 1A recommendation).[15] Screening is also recommended in first-degree relatives of patients with a AAA who are between 65 and 75 years of age, or in those older than 75 years and in good health (Grade 2C recommendation).[15] Patients older than 75 years otherwise in good health who have not been previously screened and have a history of tobacco use should also undergo a screening ultrasound examination.[15] In those with risk factors and an initial negative study, rescreening in 5 years may detect aneurysms in an additional 2%. Medicare recommends screening in males 65 to 75 years of age who have smoked at least 100 cigarettes in their lifetime or have a family history of AAA. The US Preventive Services Task Force recommends one-time screening for AAA with ultrasound examination in men aged 65 to 75 years who have ever smoked. It also recommends against routine screening for AAA with ultrasound examination in women who have never smoked and have no family history of AAA. Recommendations between societies have minimal differences, we recommend use of the extended SVS guidelines.[17]

Surveillance imaging intervals are based on the net index aortic diameter (**Table 3**). Randomized clinical trials of population screening as well as meta-analysis of these trials have demonstrated a 44% decrease in the AAA-related mortality rate in men with a statistically significant reduction in long-term (15-year) mortality with screening at risk groups. Despite these recommendations, most AAA are detected incidentally, and not on surveillance imaging.[18]

Imaging

Imaging is guided by the clinical presentation. Screening and serial monitoring can be performed with ultrasound examination. Ultrasound examination remains reliable, but is operator dependent. Serial imaging by ultrasound alone is sufficient for AAA of less than 5 cm and no suspicion for rapid growth. Ultrasound examination of the popliteal arteries is also warranted if prominent popliteal pulses are palpated on physical examination, because 20% of patients with AAA will have popliteal artery aneurysms.

If the AAA is less than 5 cm and still under surveillance, computed tomography angiography (CTA) is recommended every 3 to 6 months until reaching size for repair.[15] The initial CTA should include the chest, abdomen, and pelvis to evaluate for concomitant thoracic aneurysms. CTA also is recommended in patients with recent-onset

Table 3
Rescreening intervals for small AAAs (SVS guidelines, 2018)

Initial AAA Diameter (cm) on Screening Ultrasound Examination	Rescreening Interval
>2.5 to <3.0 cm	10 y
3.0–3.9 cm	3 y
4.0–4.9	1 y
5.0–5.4	6 mo

Data from Chaikof EL, Dalman RL, Eskandari MK, et al. The Society for Vascular Surgery practice guidelines on the care of patients with an abdominal aortic aneurysm. J Vasc Surg. 2018;67(1):2-77.e72

abdominal or back pain, particularly in the presence of a pulsatile epigastric mass or significant risk factors for AAA.[15] CTA is also indicated in those who present with peripheral thromboembolism, inflammatory or infected aneurysms, or have had increase in the size of the aneurysms of more than 5 mm in 6 months or 1 cm in a year. CTA provides data on AAA size (maximum outer wall to outer wall measurement perpendicular to the path of the aorta), morphology (size, fusiform/saccular), extent (infrarenal, juxtarenal, pararenal, suprarenal), anatomic details of renal and mesenteric vasculature (patency, location of vessels, size, angulation, branching pattern), and state of iliac/femoral outflow vessels.[19] CTA is essential for planning the details of operative or endovascular repair, along with the evaluation of other conditions like a horseshoe kidney, a retrocaval renal vein, or inflammatory changes around the aneurysm. Magnetic resonance angiography (MRA) is an option in those with genetic aortic disorders in whom lifetime cumulative dose of radiation is a concern or in those with significant renal dysfunction.

Medical management includes cholesterol reduction, antiplatelet therapy, blood pressure control, and smoking cessation. Other than smoking cessation, most other measures do not directly influence aneurysm growth, but are more relevant for the management of coexistent atherosclerotic risk factors.

Size Criteria for Repair

Elective repair of AAA is recommended in those with low or acceptable surgical risk with a fusiform AAA that is 5.5 cm or larger (Grade 1A) or in those with abdominal or back pain attributable to the aneurysm.[15,20] Repair in those with saccular aneurysms, and AAA between 5.0 cm and 5.4 cm in women, can also be considered. The SVS recommends use of the Vascular Quality Initiative perioperative mortality risk score to decide between open or endovascular aneurysm repair (EVAR)[15] The threshold of 5.5 cm was based on natural history observational studies, followed by randomized control trials comparing open or endovascular repair with surveillance.[5,21–25] The UK Small Aneurysm trial and the Aneurysm Detection and Management (ADAM) trial and a metanalysis of these studies demonstrated that repair of aneurysms of less than 5.5 cm did not improve survival for men or women of any age.[4,21,26–28] However, early repair may still be indicated in females, in younger patients, for saccular aneurysms, and for those with concomitant peripheral aneurysms or rapid expansion; these patients should specifically be referred for a vascular surgical consultation.[15,29]

Repair Options

The choice between endovascular or open surgical reconstruction is complex. It is based on AAA anatomic factors, systemic comorbidities, patient preference, follow-up plan, and life expectancy.[15] This complexity is reflected in the differences in the UK based National Institute for Health and Care Excellent guidelines recommending open repair, whereas the European Society of Vascular Surgery/SVS guidelines recommend EVAR as the treatment option in patients where both treatment modalities are possible.[20] Overall, there are 4 major randomized clinical trials that compared open AAA repair with EVAR. These were the Dutch Randomized Endovascular Aneurysm Management (DREAM),[30] Endovascular Aneurysm Repair versus Open Repair (EVAR 1),[31] Open versus Endovascular Repair (OVER),[27] and Aneurysme de l'aorte abdominale: Chirurgie versus Endoprothese (ACE) trials.[32] They all reported a significant decrease in the 30-day morbidity and mortality with EVAR, but without significant differences in long-term outcomes (**Table 4**).[33] Currently, EVAR is preferred in patients with a high perioperative risk, but open repair or EVAR may be considered for low-risk patients. In the long term, the major disadvantage of EVAR is the need for continued surveillance and reintervention. Reintervention after EVAR is required for limb occlusion or endoleaks in up to 25% of patients. Endoleaks (**Table 5**) may result in sac pressurization, aneurysm growth, and late rupture in up to 5% of patients.[34,35] There is a high rate of noncompliance (up to 60%) with follow-up programs, and those lost to follow-up have worse outcomes with an incidence of late rupture of more than 5%.[36,37] Late rupture is lower for those treated with open repair (1.4%).[38,39] Open repair requires limited follow-up, but over time patients undergoing open repair are at risk for development of incisional hernias or adhesive small bowel obstruction, a rate as high as 30%.

Follow-up

Follow-up of patients after open repair or EVAR includes a thorough history and clinical examination, pulse examination, and ankle-brachial index to rule out new-onset lower extremity claudication, ischemia, or a decrease in the ankle-brachial index suggestive of graft limb occlusion. Graft infection is a rare complication, but should be considered in those with pain, generalized sepsis, groin discharge, or anastomotic pseudoaneurysms. The SVS recommends CTA at 1 month after EVAR, and annual surveillance with either CTA or ultrasound examination.[15] Although CTA is the most sensitive, color duplex ultrasound examination is accurate in detecting type I and type III endoleaks and sac enlargement.[15] Ultrasound examination decreases the overall radiation exposure, decreases cost, and avoids the use of a nephrotoxic contrast agent. Continued surveillance with ultrasound examination is safe if CT imaging 1 year after EVAR demonstrates either no endoleak or a type II endoleak and stable sac size.[15] A repeat CTA should be obtained in patients with aneurysm sac growth greater than 5 to 10 mm in a year, a new endoleak, or graft migration.[15] CTA is also recommended at 5, 10, and 15 years after open surgical repair to identify anastomotic aneurysms or metachronous aneurysms that may occur in 1%, 5%, and 20% of patients at 5, 10, and 15 years, respectively.[40] Graft infection must be considered in any patient with

---

Table 4
Perioperative and long-term mortality after repair AAA: data from randomized controlled trials

Randomized Clinical Trial	Perioperative Mortality: EVAR vs Open Repair	Follow-up	Survival[a]: EVAR vs Open Repair	Reintervention Rate: EVAR vs Open Repair
DREAM[30]	1.2% vs 4.6%	6 y	69% vs 70%	29.6% vs 18.1%
EVAR-1[31]	1.8% vs 4.3%	12.7 y	Overall mortality 9.3 vs 8.9 deaths/100 person-years AAA-related mortality 7% vs 1% (higher incidence of late ruptures with EVAR)	Higher with EVAR
OVER[27]	0.5% vs 2.5%	14 y	68% vs 70% AAA-related mortality no difference between groups	27% vs 20%
ACE[32]	0.6% vs 1.3%	3 y	85.1% vs 82.4%	16% vs 2.4%

[a] Noted at time of last follow-up.

Table 5
Late endoleaks after EVAR

Type	Description	Incidence	Management
IA	Incomplete seal at the proximal aortic attachment site	1%–10%	Needs immediate treatment Placement of aortic cuffs, proximal graft extension, glue/coil occlusion, endoanchors, endostaples, fenestrated repairs, distal extension with iliac branch devices, consideration for open conversion
IB	Incomplete seal at the distal iliac attachment site		
IC	Inadequate seal at iliac occluder plug		
IIA	Flow from visceral vessel (lumbar, IMA, accessory, renal, hypogastric) without attachment site connection	8%–10%	Treatment necessary if persistent increase in sac size Transarterial or translumbar embolization, laparoscopic or open surgical ligation/clipping of branches
IIIA	Component separation	2%–3%	Immediate treatment necessary Relining graft
IIIB	Stent fabric disruption		
IV	Fabric porosity	Usually not a late occurrence	NA
V	Unidentified origin, endotension	1%–3%	Advanced imaging modalities to detect and reclassify/treat as types I–IV

Abbreviation: NA, not applicable.
Data from Zaiem F, Almasri J, Tello M, Prokop LJ, Chaikof EL, Murad MH. A systematic review of surveillance after endovascular aortic repair. *J Vasc Surg*. 2018;67(1):320-331.e337.

asymptomatic or rapidly increasing pseudoaneurysm, especially if there were perioperative wound healing complications. Other rare late complications like graft enteric fistulae can occur after both open and endovascular repair. These complications usually present 3 to 5 years after the procedure, with infected endografts presenting earlier than those with infected surgical grafts.[15]

VISCERAL ARTERY ANEURYSMS

Visceral artery aneurysms (VAA) are uncommon.[41] VAA represent segmental dilation of branches of the mesenteric arteries.[42] Most commonly, they are located in the splenic and hepatic arteries.[43] However, other vessels include the gastric, colic, and pancreatic arteries.[43] In some publications, renal artery aneurysms are included as VAA, but for the purpose of this review, will not be included.[44]

Incidence

VAA are rare with a prevalence of 0.01% to 0.20% according to a recent systematic review, and up to 2% based on autopsy reports.[41,43] They account for approximately 5% of all intra-abdominal aneurysms.[45] When classified according to their prevalence and anatomic location, splenic artery aneurysms are most common at 30% to 36%, and in some reports, up to 60%.[43,46] The frequency of occurrence of splenic artery aneurysms is followed by celiac artery aneurysms at 2% to 46%,[43] and hepatic artery aneurysms at 4% to 30%.[43] Aneurysms of the pancreaticoduodenal artery, superior mesenteric artery, gastroduodenal artery, gastroepiploic artery, inferior mesenteric artery, jejunal, ileal, and colic arteries are less common.[43]

Etiology of visceral artery aneurysms

Both true aneurysms and pseudoaneurysms are taken in consideration when discussing VAA.[45] In a true VAA, the vessel expands maintaining all the components of the arterial wall of at least 1.5 times its normal diameter.[43,47] Pseudoaneurysms are considered as a contained hematoma of the artery's wall.[42] True aneurysms display vessel wall disruption and adipose cell infiltration in histologic studies.[45] Other causes of true VAA include genetic conditions and connective tissue diseases such as fibromuscular dysplasia, Marfan syndrome, Ehlers–Danlos syndrome, and others.[41] Visceral artery pseudoaneurysms tend to develop after infection, trauma, local inflammation, or an iatrogenic injury that alters the structure of the vessel wall.[43,45] They tend to rupture more frequently, are more often associated with symptoms, and more frequently require emergent intervention.[44,47] VAA can occur with vasculitides such as polyarteritis nodosa and Behcet disease and other genetic disorders (eg, neurofibromatosis I).[43]

Clinical Presentation

The clinical manifestations of VAA can range from asymptomatic to potentially fatal hemodynamic instability.[47] The determinant factor is the integrity of the aneurysm wall.[47] One of 4 VAAs is diagnosed when it ruptures.[41,45] Patients with ruptured VAAs present with abdominal pain, hypotension, diaphoresis, hemobilia, hemoperitoneum, hemoretroperitoneum, gastrointestinal hemorrhage, or any sign of severe hemodynamic collapse.[45,46] The mortality rate for aneurysm ruptures ranges from 10% to 65%.[45,48] In pregnant patients with splenic or hepatic aneurysm rupture, the mortality rate is close to 100%.[5] These patients require immediate diagnosis and treatment to avoid a fatal outcome. Conversely, patients with unruptured aneurysms tend to be asymptomatic. These aneurysms tend to be diagnosed incidentally or during autopsy reports for an unrelated cause of death.[45,46,48]

Diagnosis of visceral artery aneurysms

Patients can present either with a florid clinical scenario that suggests rupture or be diagnosed incidentally through imaging.[45,48] The SVS recommends the use of CTA with 1 mm thickness sections as the preferred diagnostic tool.[45] Should CTA not be available or if concern for radiation exposure and/or chronic kidney insufficiency, MRA is an excellent second option.[45] The non–contrast-enhanced MRA is recommended for patients who have contraindications to gadolinium.[45] In emergency situations such as a possible rupture, MRA is not recommended.[46] If a ruptured visceral artery is suspected, an expedited diagnosis can be made with a multiple detector CTA with a contrast flow rate of 3 to 5 mL/s[46] Angiography can aid the surgical or procedural planning in case the CTA did not provide sufficient information.[45] The image used should provide information describing the aneurysm—specifically its size, shape, anatomic location, involved vessels, anatomic variants, concomitant aneurysms, and other information required to determine the procedural approach.[46]

Classification

VAA are classified according to their location, size, histopathology, pathology, and form.[43] Location refers to the anatomic artery (splenic and hepatic as the most common locations).[48] Size is measured as the largest diameter of the aneurysm and is considered a VAA if it is 1.5 times greater than the original size of the vessel.[46] Size is also relevant when determining treatment options.[45] Histopathologically, VAA can be separated into true aneurysms and pseudoaneurysms.[43] Pathologically, VAA are either ruptured or unruptured based on the vessel wall integrity.[43] The form/shape of the aneurysm sac could be described as saccular when bulging only to 1 side of the vessel wall or as fusiform when the dilation extends toward both sides of the arterial wall.[43]

Surveillance

The strength of the available recommendations regarding VAA surveillance is weak according to the SVS guidelines. Patients with a diagnosed VAA should be screened for other arterial aneurysms that could be present simultaneously. A recent literature study reported that 45% of 122 patients with splanchnic artery aneurysms had a concomitant aneurysm elsewhere.[49] The preferred surveillance methods are CTA, MRA, or conventional angiography, depending on patient comorbidities. Surveillance is recommended every 12 to 24 months. However, if 2 consecutive studies are stable, the interval can be spaced out to 24 to 36 months. All pseudoaneurysms and true gastric, gastroepiploic, pancreatic or duodenal, gastric, superior mesenteric, colic, and splenic aneurysms of any size in women of childbearing age should be referred to a vascular specialist. Hepatic, jejunal, ileal, and celiac aneurysms greater than 2 cm, and renal aneurysms greater than 3 cm, also require treatment.[45]

Treatment

The available treatments for VAA encompass a broad range from noninvasive clinical management to surgical procedures.[41] Indications for treatment include patients with symptoms such as embolism or rupture, aneurysms greater than 2 cm to 3 cm or twice the original artery size, growth of more than 0.5 cm per year, pseudoaneurysms, certain locations such as the duodenopancreatic arcade, pregnant or women of childbearing age, and patients who will undergo liver transplantation or who present with splenic artery aneurysms associated with portal hypertension.[41,46] As noted, treatment is suggested for patients with a higher risk of rupture whether it is due to location or size, and for patients whose mortality rate in the case of rupture is accentuated by a specific physiologic condition.[45,46] Meanwhile, patients with small asymptomatic aneurysms without factors that predispose to rupture can undergo surveillance.[45,50] Owing to the relative rarity of this condition, reports with large cohorts are scarce; thus, these recommendations must be individualized according to the patient.

Endovascular Approach

Endovascular techniques such as embolization with thrombin or other substances, coiling, and covered stents can be used for VAA.[41,43,45,51] Endovascular approaches are minimally invasive and have a shorter postoperative recovery as well as anesthesia burden.[43] Endovascular techniques are an effective option for patients whose comorbidities prevent them from undergoing open surgery.[43] Recently, Pyra and colleagues[51] reported their experience with 57 patients who underwent endovascular therapy for VAA, with 93.3% success rate. In regard to complications, 1.8% developed serious complications, characterized by a partial splenic infarction with preserved spleen function, and 10.5% developed minor complications, including hematoma and hepatic artery dissection.[51] Similarly, Martinelli and colleagues[52] report a technical success rate of 98.3% in 56 cases of VAA treated with an endovascular technique. Complications in their study occurred in 8.9% and included intestinal ischemia, aneurysm reperfusion, in-stent thrombosis, and a splenic hematoma.[52] Although endovascular treatment of VAA is feasible, it requires the availability of specific resources and carries the risk of access-related injury, embolization, and contrast-related adverse events.[43]

Open Approach

An open approach for VAA treatment allows for aneurysm ligation, excision (which enables pathologic examination), patching, primary repair, and other techniques for repair or resection.[41,43] This type of approach allows for a direct visualization of both the VAA and the organs compromised.[43] Pulli and colleagues[53] reported their 25-year experience with open surgical management of VAA in 54 patients. The mortality rate was 1.8% and major complications, which included retroperitoneal hematoma and acute pancreatitis, occurred in 3.7% of patients.[53] An open approach is used in patients whose VAA repair cannot be performed by an endovascular technique or in emergent situations that require expedited treatment.

The benefits of endovascular versus open techniques is unclear. A study from 2016 compared 56 patients with open surgery versus 57 with an endovascular approach to VAA. Survival, clinical success, intraoperative, and postoperative major complication rates were similar between the 2 groups. The treatment approach should be tailored according to the VAA characteristics and the patient's clinical history.[43,45]

SUMMARY

The identification of both abdominal aortic and VAAs is often incidental; however, screening of select populations for AAA is recommended. All symptomatic aneurysms represent a medical emergency with high morbidity; thus, prophylactic repair in the elective setting is important to minimize adverse outcomes. Atherosclerosis and its risk factors, particularly smoking, as well as inherited disorders of connective tissue, are associated with true aneurysms. Screening ultrasound examination for AAA or diagnostic imaging with CTA, MRA, and angiography are recommended in most situations and should be tailored to the patient. Management ranges from annual clinical surveillance to invasive surgical procedures with either endovascular or open surgical approaches based on individualized patient and anatomic considerations. Long-term follow-up is important to ensure repair is done when indicated or after surgery to ensure a durable repair is achieved.

CLINICS CARE POINTS

- AAA is defined as a focal abnormal increase in the diameter of the aorta, usually greater than 3 cm.

- AAAs are most common in older male smokers, but can occur in women and affect all ages. They are usually asymptomatic, and the first presentation can be with a rupture.

- Screening is recommended for adults 65 to 75 years old who have ever smoked. An underlying genetic abnormality should be suspected in younger patients with a AAA.

- Open and endovascular intervention are feasible treatment options, patients should be evaluated by a vascular surgeon for an individualized discussion of the risk–benefit ratio of the treatment plan.

- VAAs of the hepatic, splenic, and mesenteric circulation are also usually detected incidentally. Repair is indicated when these are symptomatic, saccular, or pseudoaneurysms, greater than 2 to 3 cm, especially in pregnancy or in women of childbearing age.

REFERENCES

1. Johnston KW, Rutherford RB, Tilson MD, et al. Suggested standards for reporting on arterial aneurysms. J Vasc Surg 1991;13(3):452–8.
2. Wanhainen A, Themudo R, Ahlström H, et al. Thoracic and abdominal aortic dimension in 70-year-old men and women–a population-based whole-body magnetic resonance imaging (MRI) study. J Vasc Surg 2008;47(3):504–12.
3. Gloviczki P, Pairolero P, Welch T, et al. Multiple aortic aneurysms: the results of surgical management. J Vasc Surg 1990;11(1):19–27. discussion 27-18.
4. Lederle FA, Johnson GR, Wilson SE, et al. Rupture rate of large abdominal aortic aneurysms in patients refusing or unfit for elective repair. JAMA 2002;287(22):2968–72.
5. Mortality results for randomised controlled trial of early elective surgery or ultrasonographic surveillance for small abdominal aortic aneurysms. The UK Small Aneurysm Trial Participants. Lancet 1998;352(9141):1649–55.
6. Nevitt MP, Ballard DJ, Hallett JW Jr. Prognosis of abdominal aortic aneurysms. A population-based study. N Engl J Med 1989;321(15):1009–14.
7. Scott RA, Wilson NM, Ashton HA, et al. Influence of screening on the incidence of ruptured abdominal aortic aneurysm: 5-year results of a randomized controlled study. Br J Surg 1995;82(8):1066–70.
8. Lindholt JS, Juul S, Fasting H, et al. Screening for abdominal aortic aneurysms: single centre randomised controlled trial. BMJ 2005;330(7494):750.
9. Norman PE, Jamrozik K, Lawrence-Brown MM, et al. Population based randomised controlled trial on impact of screening on mortality from abdominal aortic aneurysm. BMJ 2004;329(7477):1259.
10. Ashton HA, Buxton MJ, Day NE, et al. The Multicentre Aneurysm Screening Study (MASS) into the effect of abdominal aortic aneurysm screening on mortality in men: a randomised controlled trial. Lancet 2002;360(9345):1531–9.
11. Pleumeekers HJ, Hoes AW, van der Does E, et al. Aneurysms of the abdominal aorta in older adults. The Rotterdam Study. Am J Epidemiol 1995;142(12):1291–9.
12. Forsdahl SH, Solberg S, Singh K, et al. Abdominal aortic aneurysms, or a relatively large diameter of non-aneurysmal aortas, increase total and cardiovascular mortality: the Tromsø study. Int J Epidemiol 2010;39(1):225–32.
13. Anjum A, Powell JT. Is the incidence of abdominal aortic aneurysm declining in the 21st century? Mortality and hospital admissions for England & Wales and Scotland. Eur J Vasc Endovasc Surg 2012;43(2):161–6.
14. Brewster DC, Cronenwett JL, Hallett JW Jr, et al. Guidelines for the treatment of abdominal aortic aneurysms. Report of a subcommittee of the Joint Council of the American Association for Vascular Surgery and Society for Vascular Surgery. J Vasc Surg 2003;37(5):1106–17.
15. Chaikof EL, Dalman RL, Eskandari MK, et al. The Society for Vascular Surgery practice guidelines on the care of patients with an abdominal aortic aneurysm. J Vasc Surg 2018;67(1):2–77.e2.
16. Grootenboer N, Bosch JL, Hendriks JM, et al. Epidemiology, aetiology, risk of rupture and treatment of abdominal aortic aneurysms: does sex matter? Eur J Vasc Endovasc Surg 2009;38(3):278–84.
17. Carnevale ML, Koleilat I, Lipsitz EC, et al. Extended screening guidelines for the diagnosis of abdominal aortic aneurysm. J Vasc Surg 2020;72(6):1917–26.
18. Takagi H, Goto SN, Matsui M, et al. A further meta-analysis of population-based screening for abdominal aortic aneurysm. J Vasc Surg 2010;52(4):1103–8.
19. Smith T, Quencer KB. Best practice guidelines: imaging surveillance after endovascular aneurysm repair. AJR Am J Roentgenol 2020;214(5):1165–74.
20. Powell JT, Wanhainen A. Analysis of the differences between the ESVS 2019 and NICE 2020 guidelines for abdominal aortic aneurysm. Eur J Vasc Endovasc Surg 2020;60(1):7–15.
21. Lederle FA, Wilson SE, Johnson GR, et al. Immediate repair compared with surveillance of small abdominal aortic aneurysms. N Engl J Med 2002;346(19):1437–44.
22. Filardo G, Powell JT, Martinez MA, et al. Surgery for small asymptomatic abdominal aortic aneurysms. Cochrane Database Syst Rev 2015;2015(2):Cd001835.
23. Greenhalgh RM, Brown LC, Powell JT, et al. Endovascular repair of aortic aneurysm in patients physically ineligible for open repair. N Engl J Med 2010;362(20):1872–80.
24. Ouriel K, Clair DG, Kent KC, et al. Endovascular repair compared with surveillance for patients with small abdominal aortic aneurysms. J Vasc Surg 2010;51(5):1081–7.
25. Cao P, De Rango P, Verzini F, et al. Comparison of surveillance versus aortic endografting for small aneurysm repair (CAESAR): results from a randomised trial. Eur J Vasc Endovasc Surg 2011;41(1):13–25.
26. Lederle FA, Kane RL, MacDonald R, et al. Systematic review: repair of unruptured abdominal aortic aneurysm. Ann Intern Med 2007;146(10):735–41.

27. Lederle FA, Kyriakides TC, Stroupe KT, et al. Open versus endovascular repair of abdominal aortic aneurysm. N Engl J Med 2019;380(22):2126–35.

28. Mortality results for randomised controlled trial of early elective surgery or ultrasonographic surveillance for small abdominal aortic aneurysms. Lancet 1998;352(9141):1649–55.

29. Lo RC, Lu B, Fokkema MT, et al. Relative importance of aneurysm diameter and body size for predicting abdominal aortic aneurysm rupture in men and women. J Vasc Surg 2014;59(5):1209–16.

30. De Bruin JL, Baas AF, Buth J, et al. Long-term outcome of open or endovascular repair of abdominal aortic aneurysm. N Engl J Med 2010;362(20):1881–9.

31. Endovascular aneurysm repair versus open repair in patients with abdominal aortic aneurysm (EVAR trial 1): randomised controlled trial. Lancet 2005; 365(9478):2179–86.

32. Becquemin JP, Pillet JC, Lescalie F, et al. A randomized controlled trial of endovascular aneurysm repair versus open surgery for abdominal aortic aneurysms in low- to moderate-risk patients. J Vasc Surg 2011;53(5):1167–73.e1161.

33. Bulder RMA, Bastiaannet E, Hamming JF, et al. Meta-analysis of long-term survival after elective endovascular or open repair of abdominal aortic aneurysm. Br J Surg 2019;106(5):523–33.

34. Antoniou GA, Georgiadis GS, Antoniou SA, et al. A meta-analysis of outcomes of endovascular abdominal aortic aneurysm repair in patients with hostile and friendly neck anatomy. J Vasc Surg 2013;57(2):527–38.

35. Kouvelos GN, Oikonomou K, Antoniou GA, et al. A systematic review of proximal neck dilatation after endovascular repair for abdominal aortic aneurysm. J Endovasc Ther 2017;24(1):59–67.

36. Garg T, Baker LC, Mell MW. Adherence to postoperative surveillance guidelines after endovascular aortic aneurysm repair among Medicare beneficiaries. J Vasc Surg 2015;61(1):23–7.

37. Hicks CW, Zarkowsky DS, Bostock IC, et al. Endovascular aneurysm repair patients who are lost to follow-up have worse outcomes. J Vasc Surg 2017; 65(6):1625–35.

38. Schermerhorn ML, Buck DB, O'Malley AJ, et al. Long-term outcomes of abdominal aortic aneurysm in the Medicare population. N Engl J Med 2015; 373(4):328–38.

39. Zaiem F, Almasri J, Tello M, et al. A systematic review of surveillance after endovascular aortic repair. J Vasc Surg 2018;67(1):320–31.e337.

40. Ylönen K, Biancari F, Leo E, et al. Predictors of development of anastomotic femoral pseudoaneurysms after aortobifemoral reconstruction for abdominal aortic aneurysm. Am J Surg 2004;187(1):83–7.

41. Barrionuevo P, Malas MB, Nejim B, et al. A systematic review and meta-analysis of the management of visceral artery aneurysms. J Vasc Surg 2019;70(5):1694–9.

42. Meirelles SS. Visceral artery aneurysms. Rev Col Bras Cir 2016;43(5):311.

43. Obara H, Kentaro M, Inoue M, et al. Current management strategies for visceral artery aneurysms: an overview. Surg Today 2020;50(1):38–49.

44. van Rijn MJ, Ten Raa S, Hendriks JM, et al. Visceral aneurysms: old paradigms, new insights? Best Pract Res Clin Gastroenterol 2017;31(1):97–104.

45. Chaer RA, Abularrage CJ, Coleman DM, et al. The Society for Vascular Surgery clinical practice guidelines on the management of visceral aneurysms. J Vasc Surg 2020;72(1s):3s–39s.

46. Chiaradia M, Novelli L, Deux JF, et al. Ruptured visceral artery aneurysms. Diagn Interv Imaging 2015;96(7–8):797–806.

47. Branchi V, Meyer C, Verrel F, et al. Visceral artery aneurysms: evolving interdisciplinary management and future role of the abdominal surgeon. Eur J Med Res 2019;24(1):17.

48. Carr SC, Mahvi DM, Hoch JR, et al. Visceral artery aneurysm rupture. J Vasc Surg 2001;33(4):806–11.

49. Erben Y, Brownstein AJ, Rajaee S, et al. Natural history and management of splanchnic artery aneurysms in a single tertiary referral center. J Vasc Surg 2018;68(4):1079–87.

50. Batagini NC, El-Arousy H, Clair DG, et al. Open versus endovascular treatment of visceral artery aneurysms and pseudoaneurysms. Ann Vasc Surg 2016;35:1–8.

51. Pyra K, Szmygin M, Sojka M, et al. Endovascular treatment of visceral artery aneurysms and pseudoaneurysms - evaluation of efficacy and safety based on long-term results. Pol Przegl Chir 2019; 92(1):23–8.

52. Martinelli O, Giglio A, Irace L, et al. Single-center experience in the treatment of visceral artery aneurysms. Ann Vasc Surg 2019;60:447–54.

53. Pulli R, Dorigo W, Troisi N, et al. Surgical treatment of visceral artery aneurysms: a 25-year experience. J Vasc Surg 2008;48(2):334–42.

54. Summaries for patients. Screening for abdominal aortic aneurysm: recommendations from the U.S. Preventive Services Task Force. Ann Intern Med 2005;142(3):I52.

55. Moll FL, Powell JT, Fraedrich G, et al. Management of abdominal aortic aneurysms clinical practice guidelines of the European Society for Vascular Surgery. Eur J Vasc Endovasc Surg 2011;41(Suppl 1):S1–58.

56. Wanhainen A, Verzini F, Van Herzeele I, et al. Editor's choice - European Society for Vascular Surgery (ESVS) 2019 clinical practice guidelines on the management of abdominal aorto-iliac artery aneurysms. Eur J Vasc Endovasc Surg 2019; 57(1):8–93.

Renovascular Disease and Mesenteric Vascular Disease

Swapna Sharma, MD, MS[a], Stanislav Henkin, MD, MPH[b],
Michael N. Young, MD[b,*]

KEYWORDS

- Renal artery stenosis • Mesenteric ischemia • Fibromuscular dysplasia
- Renovascular hypertension

KEY POINTS

- The 3 clinical syndromes most often associated with renal artery stenosis (RAS) are ischemic nephropathy, renovascular hypertension, and accelerated cardiovascular disease.
- Duplex ultrasonography is the first-line screening test for most patients with suspected RAS.
- Routine endovascular or surgical intervention is not indicated for RAS, although it may be considered for patients with refractory hypertension, deterioration of renal function, recurrent "flash" pulmonary edema, or admissions for congestive heart failure.
- Acute mesenteric ischemia can be divided into 4 broad categories, including (1) arterial embolism, (2) arterial thrombosis, (3) mesenteric venous thrombosis, and (4) nonocclusive mesenteric ischemia.
- In acute mesenteric ischemia, open, endovascular, or combined hybrid revascularization should be entertained in a shared decision-making approach. In chronic mesenteric ischemia, endovascular revascularization is often the initial treatment choice.

RENAL ARTERY DISEASE
Background and Epidemiology

Renal artery stenosis (RAS) is a broad term that refers to greater than 50% narrowing of at least one renal artery or its branches causing impaired blood flow to the kidney. The most common cause of RAS is atherosclerosis, comparably affecting men and women older than 50 years.[1] Risk factors for atherosclerotic RAS include hypertension, hyperlipidemia, smoking, diabetes mellitus, and obesity. There is significant overlap between RAS and systemic atherosclerosis, including coronary artery disease (CAD) and carotid artery disease. The presence of hemodynamically significant RAS with consequent reduced glomerular filtration rate (GFR) is an independent risk factor for cardiovascular mortality.[2]

The next most common cause of RAS is fibromuscular dysplasia (FMD), which affects women more often than men and accounts for 10% of all RAS.[3,4] FMD is a segmental nonatherosclerotic, noninflammatory arterial disease that leads to stenosis of small and medium-sized arteries.[4] FMD lesions comprise a spectrum of clinical presentations, from asymptomatic and silent to hemodynamically significant with clinical manifestations of aneurysm, dissection, or occlusion.[3] Atherosclerosis affects the ostium or proximal third of the renal artery, whereas FMD is often seen in the mid or distal renal artery. The alternating regions of stenosis and dilatation form the classically described "string of beads" appearance in multifocal FMD (**Fig. 1**).[5] However, focal FMD may appear in any part of the renal artery; a physician must have a high index of suspicion—based on a

[a] The Elliot Hospital, 1 Elliot Way, Manchester, NH 03103, USA; [b] Heart and Vascular Center, Dartmouth-Hitchcock Medical Center, 1 Medical Center Drive, Lebanon, NH 03756, USA
* Corresponding author.
E-mail address: Michael.N.Young@hitchcock.org

Cardiol Clin 39 (2021) 527–537
https://doi.org/10.1016/j.ccl.2021.06.005

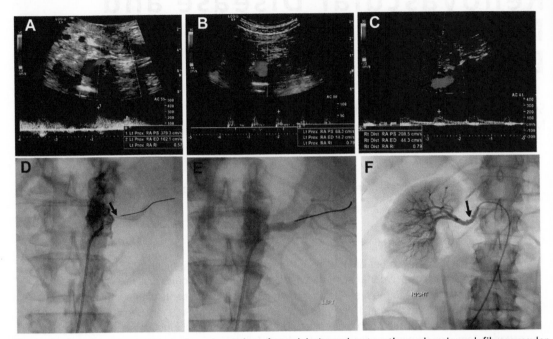

Fig. 1. Duplex ultrasonography and angiography of renal lesions due to atherosclerosis and fibromuscular dysplasia. (*A*) Duplex ultrasonography with elevated peak systolic velocity greater than 300 cm/s in proximal renal artery, consistent with hemodynamically significant renal artery stenosis. (*B*) Duplex ultrasonography after renal artery stenting showing significantly improved peak systolic velocity ~60 cm/s. (*C*) Duplex ultrasonography with elevated peak systolic velocity greater than 200 cm/s in distal renal artery, consistent with hemodynamically significant renal artery stenosis. Given location of elevated velocity, FMD was suspected as culprit. (*D*) Renal angiography showing significant ostial renal artery stenosis due to atherosclerosis (*black arrow*). (*E*) Renal angiography postdeployment of renal artery stent shows resolution of renal artery stenosis. (*F*) Renal angiography of right renal artery showing "string of beads" (*black arrow*) in midrenal artery, consistent with FMD.

combination of patient demographics and risk factor assessment—to make a correct diagnosis.[5] Other rare causes of RAS include medium vessel vasculitis, dissections, radiation, embolism, or neurofibromatosis.[4]

Determining the exact prevalence of RAS in the general population is challenging. In a population-based study of individuals aged 65 years or older, the prevalence of RAS was 6.8%, with higher prevalence in men than women.[6] As expected, the prevalence of RAS is higher in elderly patients with comorbid conditions, such as CAD, hypertension, and diabetes.[3] Atherosclerotic RAS is a progressive disease that can lead to a significant loss of kidney function in 19% to 25% of patients.[7] Progression of RAS in regard to degree of stenosis occurs at a rate of approximately 20% per year.[8] FMD is generally associated with a good prognosis and does not typically progress to complete renal artery occlusion.[4]

Pathophysiology

Hemodynamically significant RAS is defined by a reduction in 75% to 80% of the luminal area, which leads to changes in pressure gradients and reduces renal blood flow enough to stimulate renin release.[7] In the setting of a hemodynamically significant RAS, there is renal hypoperfusion that leads to local ischemia, causing microvascular damage and tubulointerstitial injury. Concurrent with this process is activation of the renin-angiotensin-aldosterone system (RAAS) (**Fig. 2**) and the plasma increase of angiotensin II levels. Angiotensin II induces transforming growth factor β, platelet-derived growth factor B, and the marcocellular protein secreted protein acidic and rich in cysteine (SPARC) by glomerular and interstitial cells.[1] These inflammatory mediators and altered cytokines lead to an increase in free radicals and oxidative stress, triggering apoptosis and necrosis. As a result of these processes, there is an augmentation of profibrotic growth factors leading to increased interstitial fibrosis (**Fig. 3**).[9]

The initial response to decreased renal blood flow is the increase in plasma renin activity and angiotensin II. Angiotensin II leads to systemic hypertension through vasoconstriction and by stimulating the release of aldosterone.

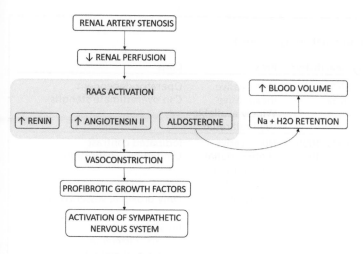

Fig. 2. Action of the renin-angiotensin-aldosterone system in renal artery stenosis.

Clinical Manifestations

There are 3 clinical syndromes most often associated with RAS—ischemic nephropathy, renovascular hypertension, and accelerated cardiovascular disease. These syndromes can occur in isolation or in various combinations.

Through autoregulation, the kidney can maintain the same GFR and renal blood flow with up to 40% reduction in renal perfusion. In ischemic nephropathy, increased oxidative stress and inflammatory cytokines lead to eventual interstitial fibrosis (see **Fig. 3**).

As renovascular hypertension progresses, there may be a need for additional antihypertensive agents to achieve a target systolic blood pressure goal of less than 130 mm Hg, as recommended for all adults.[10] RAS can also precipitate unstable angina or congestive heart failure through volume overload, peripheral arterial vasoconstriction, and direct effects of angiotensin on the myocardium.[4] An acute increase in left ventricular end diastolic pressure is the substrate for flash pulmonary edema; this may occur in the setting of unilateral or more commonly, bilateral RAS, during which there is impaired natriuresis.[11]

Diagnosis

Early detection and treatment of renovascular disease can improve hypertension and potentially prevent progressive renal insufficiency.[12] The 2017 European Society of Cardiology Guidelines recommend duplex ultrasonography of the renal arteries as the first-line noninvasive imaging modality, followed by computed tomographic (CT) angiography (CTA) or magnetic resonance angiography (MRA).[13] However, if these tests are inconclusive and there is a high suspicion for RAS, diagnostic angiography is suggested. A summary of the advantages and disadvantages of these methods is presented in **Table 1**.

Duplex imaging is noninvasive, well tolerated by patients, inexpensive, and widely available; it is the test of choice in patients with renal insufficiency and suspicion for RAS. Stenosis greater than 50% is defined by elevated renal artery peak systolic velocity (PSV, usually >200 cm/s) and/or ratio of renal artery PSV to perirenal aortic systolic velocity greater than 3.5.[14] Screening for FMD with duplex ultrasonography should only be done in specialized centers with high FMD volume, because FMD can be mistaken for other conditions that cause elevated velocities, such as atherosclerosis or dissection.[5] Combining velocity criteria with two-dimensional B-mode evaluation (evidence of vessel tortuosity and/or aneurysm) improves the accuracy of FMD diagnosing.[15] If FMD is suspected, the degree of stenosis should not be reported because this cannot be accurately determined in multifocal FMD.[16] The peak cutoffs

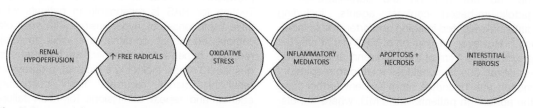

Fig. 3. Proposed fibrogenic pathways leading to renal parenchymal injury.

Table 1
Summary of methods for diagnosis of renal artery stenosis

Diagnostic test	Sensitivity/specificity[32]	Pros	Cons
Duplex ultrasonography	Sensitivity 85% Specificity 92%	Noninvasive Inexpensive Widely available Well tolerated	Operator dependent Can overestimate stenosis
Computed tomography angiography	Sensitivity 89%–100% Specificity 82%–100%	Noninvasive Higher spatial resolution Less artifact	Iodinated contrast Limited by calcification
Magnetic resonance angiography	Sensitivity 96% Specificity 93%	Less nephrotoxic	Only proximal vessel visible
Digital subtraction angiography		Gold standard	Invasive Arterial dissection Cholesterol emboli Contrast-induced nephrotoxicity Catheter-related complications

for renal artery ratio and PSV, among other cutoffs, should be subject to internal validation within an accredited vascular laboratory. Renal duplex ultrasonography is the modality of choice to assess for renal patency after surgical or endovascular repair.[17] However, compared with angiography, duplex ultrasonography generally overestimates the degree of stenosis.[18]

CTA is noninvasive, technically easier to perform than MRA, and provides multiplanar visualization of the renal arterial anatomy.[19] However, it requires iodinated contrast and should not be used for patients who have significant renal insufficiency. CTA has a higher spatial resolution and less artifact compared with MRA, although calcification of the vessel wall can make visualization of the degree of stenosis challenging. CTA is the test of choice for diagnosis of FMD due to better spatial resolution.[4]

MRA is an imaging option that may be used as a screening test in high-risk patients with renal insufficiency. Although administration of older gadolinium agents was associated with up to 5% incidence of nephrogenic systemic fibrosis (NSF) in patients with severe renal failure, newer gadolinium agents have much lower risk of NSF.[20,21] In addition, there are several renal MRA techniques that do not rely on the administration of gadolinium-based contrast agents, including diffusion-weighted imaging and arterial spin labeling.[22] However, a limitation of MRA is that only the proximal 3 to 4 cm of the main renal artery can be visualized due to signal loss related to respiratory motion that becomes more evident further from the aorta.[23] In patients with FMD, where the disease more commonly affects the mid and distal

renal arteries, this may be of greater relevance with regard to the diagnostic evaluation.

Catheter angiography is accepted as the gold standard for the diagnosis of RAS. Intravascular digital subtraction angiography is performed if noninvasive tests remain inconclusive. The limitations include exposure to contrast media, risk of arterial dissection or cholesterol embolization, bleeding, sedation, and radiation exposure. However, conventional angiography offers the benefit of possible therapeutic intervention with balloon angioplasty or stenting at the time of diagnosis. In patients who are at exceedingly high risk of contrast nephropathy, carbon dioxide angiography is an effective alternative to iodinated contrast medium in imaging patients with peripheral artery disease while preserving renal function.[24]

WHO TO SCREEN?

Most hypertension is not due to RAS but rather essential hypertension. RAS is present in less than 1% of patients with mild hypertension, but its prevalence increases up to 40% in patients with severe or refractory hypertension.[25] As such, it is not cost effective to offer widespread testing given the low prevalence of RAS in the general population. Testing for RAS is reasonable in patients who have rapid onset of hypertension (<40 year old) without additional cardiovascular risk factors), resistant hypertension (defined as hypertension despite >3 drugs, including a diuretic), progressive renal insufficiency, recurrent "flash" pulmonary edema, and repeat admissions for heart failure despite preserved left ventricular function.[12,26]

Management

Atherosclerotic renal artery stenosis

Management strategies for RAS include both medical therapies and revascularization. Medical therapy is critical in these patients, because they often have systemic atherosclerosis that confers added morbidity. The mainstay of medical treatment includes aggressive secondary risk factor modification—lipid reduction with high intensity statin, antiplatelet therapy with low-dose aspirin, strict glucose control, smoking cessation, and control of hypertension. Angiotensin-converting enzyme inhibitors (ACEIs) or angiotensin receptor blockers (ARBs) are both effective means of blood pressure reduction by targeting the RAAS.

The goal of renal artery revascularization is to improve renal blood flow by reducing obstruction to renal perfusion with the goal of stabilizing or restoring renal function. Revascularization options include percutaneous transluminal renal artery angioplasty (PTA), renal artery stenting, or surgical bypass.[27] PTA had largely replaced surgical revascularization in the 1900s due to trials showing similar efficacy and need for fewer antihypertensives after PTA.[28,29] PTA has several associated risks, including bleeding, catheter-related complications, contrast-induced nephropathy, arterial dissection, and cholesterol emboli.

A summary of clinical trials, their outcomes, and limitations is shown in **Table 2**. The Cardiovascular Outcomes in Renal Atherosclerotic Lesions trial demonstrated that patients with RAS had no improvement in outcomes with the addition of renal artery stenting to medical therapy.[30] Multiple other clinical trials showed that routine renal artery stenting is not superior to medical therapy and therefore should be reserved for patients with progressive renal dysfunction or uncontrolled hypertension despite medical therapy, or in cases of flash pulmonary edema/heart failure.[31] Although renal artery stenting may not improve renal function, it can stabilize GFR or delay time to renal replacement therapy.[32–34]

Per the 2018 American College of Cardiology/American Heart Association/Society for Cardiovascular Angiography & Interventions/Society of Interventional Radiology/Society of Vascular Medicine Appropriate Use Criteria, in the case of hemodynamically significant RAS (70%–99% stenosis or 50%–69% stenosis with resting translesional gradient >20 mm Hg with hemodynamic significance), medical therapy is the mainstay of treatment in patients with unilateral atrophic kidney (<7 cm pole to pole) or accelerating decline in renal function in the setting of unilateral RAS. Renal artery stenting is recommended in patients with accelerated decline in renal function in the setting of bilateral RAS or a solitary viable kidney with RAS.[35]

Fibromuscular dysplasia

Patients with FMD should receive appropriate medical therapies (aspirin and/or control of hypertension), undergo surveillance of affected vasculature, and proceed with revascularization if hypertension is not controlled with medications alone.[5] Patients who have incidental FMD and are normotensive can continue with aspirin alone. Patients with FMD often have essential or renovascular hypertension associated with renal artery involvement, for which ACEI and ARB are recommended.[5]

Patients with FMD who are hypertensive despite medical therapy or with progressive renal insufficiency may benefit from revascularization with PTA.[4] Endovascular stenting should be avoided because of risk of arterial dissection, stent fracture, in-stent thrombosis, migration, and aneurysm formation.[36] Surgical revascularization is reserved for patients with complex disease not amenable to PTA.

Clinics care points

- The most common cause of RAS is atherosclerosis.
- The 3 clinical syndromes most often associated with RAS are ischemic nephropathy, renovascular hypertension, and accelerated cardiovascular disease.
- Routine screening for RAS is not recommended but is reasonable in patients who have rapid onset of hypertension, resistant hypertension, progressive renal insufficiency, recurrent pulmonary edema, or repeat admissions for heart failure.
- Duplex ultrasonography is the first-line screening test for most patients.
- Routine endovascular or surgical intervention is not indicated for RAS, although it may be considered for patients with refractory hypertension, recurrent "flash" pulmonary edema, or admissions for congestive heart failure.

MESENTERIC ARTERY DISEASE
Background and Epidemiology

Acute mesenteric ischemia (AMI) and chronic mesenteric ischemia (CMI) have varied causes and presentations. AMI is most often caused by acute arterial obstruction (ie, in the case of mesenteric arterial or venous thrombosis or embolism) but can also occur without arterial obstruction in low-flow states. CMI is most often caused by arterial obstruction, typically in a setting of progressive atherosclerosis. CMI is associated with high rates

Table 2
Summary of major randomized controlled trials examining treatment options in renal artery stenosis

Trial	Year	Intervention	N	Average age (y) [range]	% Male	eGFR (mL/min/1.73 m²) [range]	Mean renal stenosis % [range]	SBP (mm Hg) [range]	Primary outcome	Secondary outcomes	Median follow-up (mo)	Results	Weaknesses
STAR[35]	2009	1	140	67	45	46	-	163	Renal function (20% or greater decrease in CrCl)	Procedural complications, changes in BP, refractory or malignant HTN, CV mortality, all-cause mortality	24	• Improvement in BP in both arms but no difference between groups • No difference in progression of renal failure • Significant stent-related complications	• Small sample size and underpowered • Excluded patients with resistant HTN
		1 + 2		66	43	45	-	160					
ASTRAL[56]	2009	1	806	71 [43–88]	63.0	39.8 [7.1–121.7]	75 [20–99]	152 [90–241]	Renal function (reciprocal of sCr)	1. Blood pressure 2. Time to renal and major CV events 3. Mortality	34	• No improvement in blood pressure or reduction in renal or CV events or mortality	• Severity of RAS not confirmed • Cr concentration used as indirect measure of GFR
		1 + (2 or 3)		70 [42–86]	63.0	40.3 [5.4–124.5]	76 [40–100]	149 [87–270]					
CORAL[33]	2014	1	947	69.0 ± 9.0	48.9	57.4 ± 21.7	74.3 ± 13.1	150.4 ± 23.0	Major[a] CV or renal event	Individual components of primary end point and all-cause mortality	43	• No reduction in renal or CV events • No difference in all-cause mortality	• High-risk patients less likely referred • Did not include patients with FMD
		1 + 2		69.3 ± 9.4	51.0	58.0 ± 23.4	72.5 ± 14.6	149.9 ± 23.2					

Intervention: 1, medical therapy; 2, PTA/stent; 3, surgical revascularization.

Abbreviations: ASTRAL, Angioplasty and Stenting for Renal Artery Lesions; BP, blood pressure; CORAL, Cardiovascular Outcomes in Renal Atherosclerotic Lesions; CrCl, creatinine clearance; CV, cardiovascular; eGFR, estimated glomerular filtration rate; HTN, hypertension; PTA, percutaneous transluminal renal artery angioplasty; STAR, Stent Placement in Patients with Atherosclerotic Renal Artery Stenosis and Impaired Renal Function.

of morbidity and mortality, although it is often underdiagnosed and the true incidence of CMI is unknown.[37] Symptomatic AMI accounts for less than 1 of every 1000 hospital admissions.[38] Mesenteric ischemia affects more women than men, with a median age of 70 years.[39,40]

Pathophysiology

Acute mesenteric artery occlusion

The celiac artery (CA), superior mesenteric artery (SMA), and inferior mesenteric artery (IMA) are the 3 major vessels of the gut. The CA supplies the foregut (esophagus to midduodenum), the SMA supplies the midgut (midduodenum to midtransverse colon), and the IMA supplies the hindgut (midtransverse colon to rectum). There is an extensive collateral system that protects against transient periods of hypoperfusion. The watershed regions that lay between these arteries are prone to ischemia and include the splenic flexure and the rectosigmoid junction.

The causes of AMI can be divided into 4 broad categories: (1) arterial embolism, (2) arterial thrombosis, (3) mesenteric venous thrombosis (MVT), and (4) nonocclusive mesenteric ischemia (NOMI). Ischemia leads to infarction, typically from the mucosa outward, followed by perforation, peritoneal irritation, bowel necrosis, lactic acidosis, and death. AMI from embolism is more common than from thrombosis.[39] Arterial emboli most typically lodge at a narrowing distal to the origin of a major branch, such as the takeoff of the middle colic artery. The anatomy of the SMA, with a narrow takeoff angle from the aorta, makes this visceral vessel most susceptible to emboli. In contrast, the IMA is less often affected due to its small caliber. Etiologies of emboli include left ventricular mural thrombus, atrial fibrillation, atrial thrombi in mitral stenosis, paradoxic emboli across an interatrial septal defect, or septic emboli from endocarditis.[41]

Arterial thrombosis most often occurs at points of severe atherosclerotic narrowing.[42] Risk factors that can contribute to thrombosis include low cardiac output, dehydration, and hypercoagulable states (ie, recent surgery or prothrombotic disorders, such as antiphospholipid antibody syndrome).[43,44] Patients with atherosclerosis often develop collateral blood flow that delays presentation.

MVT may occur due to vessel damage (direct vessel injury, pancreatitis, or diverticulitis), local venous stasis, or thrombophilia.[39] MVT is often associated with cirrhosis or portal hypertension, malignancy, and oral contraceptive use. Many of these patients have a history of other venous thromboembolism, such as a deep vein thrombosis or pulmonary embolism.[38]

NOMI occurs in the absence of thrombosis or embolism when there is inadequate blood supply to perfuse the bowel. MVT is most likely to occur in low-flow states, such as critical illness in septic or cardiogenic shock, and is exacerbated by the presence of atherosclerosis. Other risk factors for NOMI include the use of vasoconstrictor substances, such as vasopressors and cocaine, which can functionally worsen existing regions of stenosis.[38]

Chronic mesenteric ischemia

CMI is a long-standing process often associated with weight loss and chronic postprandial abdominal pain. The latter, referred to as abdominal angina, is accompanied by a fear of eating. The risk factors for CMI are similar to that of atherosclerosis, including hyperlipidemia, hypertension, obesity, and diabetes.[45] Most often, CMI is caused by atherosclerosis, but can also be seen in several nonatherosclerotic conditions, including neurofibromatosis, vasculitides, radiation injury, and medial arcuate ligament compression, among others.[33,46] Given the range of causes for chronic abdominal pain, the diagnosis of mesenteric ischemia is often delayed despite a battery of tests being performed, such as upper endoscopy, abdominal computed tomography, or ultrasonography.

Clinical Manifestations

Patients with AMI often present with abdominal pain due to peritoneal irritation that is "out of proportion" to the physical examination. Many of the patients with AMI have preexisting vascular disease, in whom AMI may be a severe consequence of CMI. Patients with CMI often have had years of unexplained weight loss, food aversion, physical wasting, failure to thrive, and chronic abdominal pain. An abdominal bruit may be appreciated with auscultation.

Diagnosis

The diagnosis of mesenteric ischemia is a clinical one, supported by presenting symptoms, history, and imaging. Duplex ultrasonography is a noninvasive, widely available modality that can aid in the identification of arterial stenosis or occlusion or mesenteric venous thrombosis. Duplex ultrasonography has an overall accuracy of 90% for the detection of stenoses that are greater than 70% in diameter or occlusions of the celiac or superior mesenteric arteries.[42] Ultrasonography can be useful in detecting larger thrombi in MVT but can miss thrombus in small vessels.[43] This technique is highly operator dependent and is also limited by patient habitus and clinical condition. If possible, patients should remain fasting before a full ultrasonographic study, to optimize the quality of the imaging.

Per the 2020 Clinical Practice Guidelines from the Society of Vascular Surgery, patients who are symptomatic with CMI should undergo an expedited workup, including CTA.[47] Catheter-based angiography is the gold standard for the diagnosis of mesenteric ischemia, but the advent of high-resolution CT has improved the ability to diagnose mesenteric ischemia in a timely way. CTA can visualize sites of atherosclerotic lesions. If a patient has an unclear degree of stenosis with duplex ultrasonography or CTA, catheter angiography can be performed to provide a definitive diagnosis. The arteriographic sign of proximal mesenteric arterial obstruction is an enlarged "arc of Riolan," or the "meandering mesenteric artery," which refers to the collateral vessel that connects the left colic branch of the IMA with the SMA.[42] Lateral views are preferred to provide visualization of proximal disease, and anterior views are helpful in diagnosing ischemia in distal vessels (**Fig. 4**).[39]

Treatment

Acute mesenteric ischemia

Initial medical therapy for AMI includes fluid resuscitation, correction of electrolyte abnormalities, and hemodynamic monitoring. It is important to avoid vasoconstrictors that may exacerbate ischemia and induce vasospasm. Given the accompanying bacterial translocation, antibiotics

are warranted. Intravenous anticoagulation is recommended in arterial thrombosis to prevent the propagation of thrombus.[44] AMI is a surgical emergency and often requires emergent exploratory laparotomy to investigate the extent of bowel necrosis and to perform bowel resection, if necessary. If a patient requires a bowel resection, mortality can be as high as 80%.[48] Revascularization may be achieved through endovascular therapies, surgical bypass, or hybrid intervention.[49] If possible, endovascular therapy should be the procedure of choice because it is associated with lower rates of mortality and unnecessary bowel resection.[50,51] In cases of septic shock and peritonitis, open surgery is almost always necessary. In addition, a "second look" laparotomy may be necessary after endovascular intervention is complete to inspect the bowel.[52]

MVT without evidence of bowel necrosis can be managed nonoperatively with the early use of anticoagulation. Still, some patients ultimately require bowel resection.[42]

Chronic mesenteric ischemia

In the case of asymptomatic CMI, prophylactic revascularization is unnecessary. However, in symptomatic CMI, revascularization (with SMA as the primary target) should not be delayed.[53] Endovascular repair is associated with significant clinical success and decreased morbidity and mortality when compared with open surgical bypass.[52] As such, endovascular repair with a balloon-expandable covered intraluminal stent is recommended as the first-line treatment for CMI.

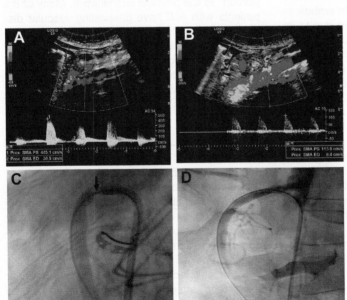

Fig. 4. Representative images of chronic mesenteric ischemia in the setting of hemodynamically significant superior mesenteric artery (SMA) stenosis. (*A*) Duplex ultrasonography shows elevated peak systolic velocity greater than 400 cm/s of proximal SMA, suggesting hemodynamically significant SMA stenosis. (*B*) Duplex ultrasonography shows significantly improved peak systolic velocity ~100 cm/s after SMA stenting. (*C*) SMA angiography shows ostial SMA stenosis (*black arrow*). (*D*) Resolution of SMA stenosis after stent deployment.

Covered stents have been shown to be associated with fewer stenoses, recurrences, and reinterventions than bare metal stents in patients undergoing primary intervention for CMI.[54] Open surgical revascularization should be reserved for patients with lesions not amenable to endovascular repair, and younger patients who may have long-term benefits that outweigh the perioperative risks should be selected.[53] Long-term follow-up and annual surveillance with mesenteric duplex ultrasonography is recommended after revascularization.[53] Risk factor medication with antiplatelet therapy, high-intensity statin, and blood pressure control are important, before and after revascularization.[53,55]

CLINICS CARE POINTS

- CMI is most often caused by arterial obstruction, typically in a setting of progressive atherosclerosis.

- The causes of AMI can be divided into four broad categories, including (1) arterial embolism, (2) arterial thrombosis, (3) MVT, and (4) NOMI.

- Patients with AMI often present with acute onset of pain "out of proportion" to physical examination, whereas patients with CMI often have years of food aversion, failure to thrive, and chronic abdominal pain.

- Duplex ultrasonography or CTA are the screening tests of choice for CMI, whereas angiography is the gold-standard modality.

- AMI often requires emergent exploratory laparotomy to investigate the extent of bowel necrosis and to perform bowel resection if necessary. In CMI, endovascular revascularization is most often the initial treatment of choice.

DISCLOSURE

The authors have nothing to disclose.

REFERENCES

1. Carmichael P, Carmichael AR. Atherosclerotic renal artery stenosis: from diagnosis to treatment. Postgrad Med J 1999;75(887):527–36.

2. Chonchol M, Linas S. Diagnosis and management of ischemic nephropathy. Clin J Am Soc Nephrol 2006; 1(2):172–81.

3. Olin JW, Sealove BA. Diagnosis, management, and future developments of fibromuscular dysplasia. J Vasc Surg 2011;53(3):826–36.

4. Weber BR, Dieter RS. Renal artery stenosis: epidemiology and treatment. Int J Nephrol Renovascular Dis 2014;7:169.

5. Gornik HL, Persu A, Adlam D, et al. First international consensus on the diagnosis and management of fibromuscular dysplasia. Vasc Med 2019;24(2):164–89.

6. Hansen KJ, Edwards MS, Craven TE, et al. Prevalence of renovascular disease in the elderly: a population-based study. J Vasc Surg 2002;36(3): 443–51.

7. Simon G. What is critical renal artery stenosis? Implications for treatment. Am J Hypertens 2000;13(11): 1189–93.

8. Zierler RE, Bergelin RO, Isaacson JA, et al. Natural history of atherosclerotic renal artery stenosis: a prospective study with duplex ultrasonography. J Vasc Surg 1994;19(2):250–8.

9. Textor SC. Ischemic nephropathy: where are we now? J Am Soc Nephrol 2004;15(8):1974–82.

10. Whelton PK, Carey RM, Aronow WS, et al. 2017 ACC/AHA/AAPA/ABC/ACPM/AGS/APhA/ASH/ ASPC/NMA/PCNA guideline for the prevention, detection, evaluation, and management of high blood pressure in adults: a report of the American College of Cardiology/American Heart Association Task Force on Clinical Practice Guidelines. J Am Coll Cardiol 2018;71(19):e127–248.

11. Pickering T, Devereux R, James G, et al. Recurrent pulmonary oedema in hypertension due to bilateral renal artery stenosis: treatment by angioplasty or surgical revascularisation. Lancet 1988;332(8610): 551–2.

12. Beutler JJ, Ampting van JMA, Ven van de PJG, et al. Long-term effects of arterial stenting on kidney function for patients with ostial atherosclerotic renal artery stenosis and renal insufficiency. J Am Soc Nephrol 2001;12:1475–81.

13. Aboyans V, Ricco JB, Bartelink MLE, et al. 2017 ESC guidelines on the diagnosis and treatment of peripheral arterial diseases, in collaboration with the European Society for vascular surgery (ESVS) Document covering atherosclerotic disease of extracranial carotid and vertebral, mesenteric, renal, upper and lower extremity arteries Endorsed by: the European stroke Organization (ESO) the Task Force for the diagnosis and treatment of peripheral arterial diseases of the European Society of Cardiology (ESC) and of the European Society for vascular. Eur Heart J 2018;39(9):763–816.

14. Granata A, Fiorini F, Andrulli S, et al. Doppler ultrasound and renal artery stenosis: an overview. J Ultrasound 2009;12(4):133–43.

15. Lewis S, Kadian-Dodov D, Bansal A, et al. Multimodality imaging of fibromuscular dysplasia. Abdom Radiol 2016;41(10):2048–60.

16. Olin JW, Gornik HL, Bacharach JM, et al. Fibromuscular dysplasia: state of the science and critical

unanswered questions: a scientific statement from the American Heart Association. Circulation 2014; 129(9):1048–78.

17. Hudspeth DA, Hansen KJ, Reavis SW, et al. Renal duplex sonography after treatment of renovascular disease. J Vasc Surg 1993;18(3):381–90.

18. Drieghe B, Madaric J, Sarno G, et al. Assessment of renal artery stenosis: side-by-side comparison of angiography and duplex ultrasound with pressure gradient measurements. Eur Heart J 2008;29(4): 517–24.

19. Zhang H, Prince MR. Improving Interpretation of MRA and CTA in patients with suspected renal artery stenosis. Vascular Disease Manag 2011;8: E34–7.

20. Soloff EV, Wang CL. Safety of gadolinium-based contrast agents in patients with stage 4 and 5 chronic kidney disease: a Radiologist's Perspective. Kidney360 2020;1(2):123–6.

21. Al-Katib S, Shetty M, Jafri SMA, et al. Radiologic assessment of native renal vasculature: a multimodality review. Radiographics 2017;37(1): 136–56.

22. Roditi G, Maki JH, Oliveira G, et al. Renovascular imaging in the NSF Era. J Magn Reson Imaging 2009; 30(6):1323–34.

23. Tan KT, Van Beek EJR, Brown PWG, et al. Magnetic resonance angiography for the diagnosis of renal artery stenosis: a meta-analysis. Clin Radiol 2002; 57(7):617–24.

24. Gupta A, Dosekun AK, Kumar V. Carbon dioxide-angiography for patients with peripheral arterial disease at risk of contrast-induced nephropathy. World J Cardiol 2020;12(2):76.

25. Bokhari MR, Bokhari SRA. Renal artery stenosis. In: StatPearls. Treasure Island (FL): StatPearls Publishing; 2021.

26. Jennings CG, Houston JG, Severn A, et al. Renal artery stenosis—when to screen, what to stent? Curr Atheroscler Rep 2014;16(6):416.

27. Mousa AY, AbuRahma AF, Bozzay J, et al. Update on intervention versus medical therapy for atherosclerotic renal artery stenosis. J Vasc Surg 2015; 61(6):1613–23.

28. Weibull H, Bergqvist D, Bergentz SE, et al. Percutaneous transluminal renal angioplasty versus surgical reconstruction of atherosclerotic renal artery stenosis: a prospective randomized study. J Vasc Surg 1993;18(5):841–52.

29. Dorros G, Jaff M, Mathiak L, et al. Multicenter Palmaz stent renal artery stenosis revascularization registry report: four-year follow-up of 1,058 successful patients. Catheter Cardiovasc Interv 2002;55(2): 182–8.

30. Gupta R, Assiri S, Cooper CJ. Renal artery stenosis: new findings from the CORAL trial. Curr Cardiol Rep 2017;19(9):1–6.

31. Creager M, Loscalzo J, Beckman JA. Vascular Medicine: A companion to Braunwald's heart disease. Boston (MA): Elsevier Health Sciences; 2012.

32. Cooper CJ, Murphy TP, Cutlip DE, et al. Stenting and medical therapy for atherosclerotic renal-artery stenosis. N Engl J Med 2014;370(1):13–22.

33. Bavry AA. Angioplasty and stenting for renal artery lesions (ASTRAL). Chicago (IL): SCAI-ACC i2 Summit/ACC; 2008.

34. Bax L, Woittiez AJJ, Kouwenberg HJ, et al. Stent placement in patients with atherosclerotic renal artery stenosis and impaired renal function: a randomized trial. Ann Intern Med 2009;150(12):840–8.

35. Bailey SR, Beckman JA, Dao TD, et al. ACC/AHA/SCAI/SIR/SVM 2018 appropriate use criteria for peripheral artery intervention: a report of the American college of cardiology appropriate use criteria task force, American heart association, society for cardiovascular angiography and interventions, society of interventional radiology, and society for vascular medicine. J Am Coll Cardiol 2019;73(2):214–37.

36. Wang LC, Scott DJ, Clemens MS, et al. Mechanism of stent failure in a patient with fibromuscular dysplasia following renal artery stenting. Ann Vasc Surg 2015;29(1):123.e19.

37. Herbert GS, Steele SR. Acute and chronic mesenteric ischemia. Surg Clin North Am 2007;87(5): 1115–34.

38. Clair DG, Beach JM. Mesenteric ischemia. N Engl J Med 2016;374(10):959–68.

39. Sidawy AN, Perler BA. Rutherford's vascular surgery and endovascular therapy, E-Book. Philadelphia: Elsevier Health Sciences; 2018.

40. Hirsch AT, Haskal ZJ, Hertzer NR, et al. ACC/AHA 2005 practice guidelines for the management of patients with peripheral arterial disease (lower extremity, renal, mesenteric, and abdominal aortic) a collaborative report from the American Association for Vascular Surgery/Society for Vascular Surgery,* Society for Cardiovascular Angiography and Interventions, Society for Vascular Medicine and Biology, Society of Interventional Radiology, and the ACC/AHA Task Force on Practice Guidelines (writing committee to develop guidelines for the management. Circulation 2006;113(11):e463–654.

41. Mastoraki A, Mastoraki S, Tziava E, et al. Mesenteric ischemia: pathogenesis and challenging diagnostic and therapeutic modalities. World J Gastrointest Pathophysiol 2016;7(1):125.

42. Acosta S. Mesenteric ischemia. Curr Opin Crit Care 2015;21(2):171–8.

43. Russell CE, Wadhera RK, Gregory P. Mesenteric venous thrombosis. Circulation 2015;131(18): 1599–603.

44. Falkensammer J, Oldenburg WA. Surgical and medical management of mesenteric ischemia. Curr Treat Options Cardiovasc Med 2006;8(2):137–43.

45. Oderich GS. Current concepts in the management of chronic mesenteric ischemia. Curr Treat Options Cardiovasc Med 2010;12(2):117–30.

46. Oderich GS, Sullivan TM, Bower TC, et al. Vascular abnormalities in patients with neurofibromatosis syndrome type I: clinical spectrum, management, and results. J Vasc Surg 2007;46(3):475–84.

47. Huber TS, Bjorck M, Chandra A, et al, Evidence Review Committee. Chronic mesenteric ischemia clinical practice guideline from the Society for vascular surgery. J Vasc Surg 2020;73(1S): 87S–115S.

48. Jrvinen O, Laurikka J, Salenius JP, et al. January). Acute intestinal ischaemia. A review of 214 cases. Ann chirurgiae gynaecologiae 1994;83(No. 1):22–5.

49. Wyers MC, Powell RJ, Nolan BW, et al. Retrograde mesenteric stenting during laparotomy for acute occlusive mesenteric ischemia. J Vasc Surg 2007; 45(2):269–75.

50. Beaulieu RJ, Arnaoutakis KD, Abularrage CJ, et al. Comparison of open and endovascular treatment of acute mesenteric ischemia. J Vasc Surg 2014; 59(1):159–64.

51. Block TA, Acosta S, Björck M. Endovascular and open surgery for acute occlusion of the superior mesenteric artery. J Vasc Surg 2010;52(4):959–66.

52. Hohenwalter EJ. Chronic mesenteric ischemia: diagnosis and treatment. Semin Intervent Radiol 2009; 26(4):345–51. https://doi.org/10.1055/s-0029-1242198.

53. Tendera M, Aboyans V, Bartelink ML, et al. European Stroke Organisation; ESC Committee for Practice Guidelines. ESC Guidelines on the diagnosis and treatment of peripheral artery diseases: Document covering atherosclerotic disease of extracranial carotid and vertebral, mesenteric, renal, upper and lower extremity arteries: the Task Force on the Diagnosis and Treatment of Peripheral Artery Diseases of the European Society of Cardiology (ESC). Eur Heart J 2011;32(22):2851–906.

54. Oderich GS, Erdoes LS, LeSar C, et al. Comparison of covered stents versus bare metal stents for treatment of chronic atherosclerotic mesenteric arterial disease. J Vasc Surg 2013;58(5):1316–24.

55. Capell WH, Bonaca MP, Nehler MR, et al. Rationale and design for the Vascular Outcomes study of ASA along with rivaroxaban in endovascular or surgical limb revascularization for peripheral artery disease (VOYAGER PAD). Am Heart J 2018;199:83–91.

56. Mistry S, Ives N, Harding J, et al. Angioplasty and STent for Renal Artery Lesions (ASTRAL trial): rationale, methods and results so far. J Hum Hypertens 2007;21(7):511–5.

Risk Stratification and Management of Extracranial Carotid Artery Disease

Anna K. Krawisz, MD[a,b,c], Brett J. Carroll, MD[b,c],
Eric A. Secemsky, MD, MSc[a,b,c],*

KEYWORDS

- Carotid artery stenosis • Stroke • Atherosclerosis • Carotid endarterectomy
- Carotid artery stenting

KEY POINTS

- Stroke and transient ischemic attack (TIA) caused by carotid stenosis are associated with a high rate of recurrence of stroke.
- All patients with carotid artery disease should be treated with optimal medical therapy.
- Revascularization is not recommended for a complete carotid occlusion or patients with less than 50% stenosis.
- A risk-benefit assessment should be performed to determine whether revascularization should be recommended for a given patient. This should include the degree of carotid stenosis, presence or absence of symptoms attributable to the carotid lesion, and perioperative risk.

INTRODUCTION

Stroke is the fifth leading cause of death in the United States and the second leading cause of death worldwide.[1,2] Stroke causes significant disability and reduced quality of life, and is responsible for a large burden of health care expenditures. Extracranial carotid artery disease is a leading cause of stroke, causing 8% to 15% of ischemic strokes.[3,4] There are high rates of recurrence for stroke and transient ischemic attack (TIA) caused by carotid artery stenosis.[5] It is essential that patients with carotid artery disease be treated with optimal medical therapy and appropriate revascularization strategies, when indicated, to prevent first-time and repeat strokes.

Carotid artery stenosis is typically diagnosed via four imaging modalities: invasive cerebral angiography, carotid duplex ultrasound (CDUS), magnetic resonance angiography (MRA), and computed tomographic angiography (CTA). Although invasive cerebral angiography is the gold standard for diagnosis, noninvasive imaging techniques are used more commonly to avoid the risk of complications. CDUS is recommended for the initial evaluation of suspected carotid artery stenosis.[6] CDUS, MRA, and CTA have high

Funding: Dr E. Secemsky is supported by NIH/NHLBI K23HL150290 and Harvard Medical School's Shore Faculty Development Award.

Relationships with Industry: E. Secemsky: Consulting/Scientific Advisory Board: Abbott, Bayer, BD, Boston Scientific, Cook, CSI, Inari, Janssen, Medtronic, Philips, and Venture Medical.; Research Grants: AstraZeneca, BD, Boston Scientific, Cook, CSI, Laminate Medical, Medtronic, and Philips. All other authors have nothing to disclose.

[a] Richard A. and Susan F. Smith Center for Outcomes Research in Cardiology, Division of Cardiology, Department of Medicine, Beth Israel Deaconess Medical Center, 375 Longwood Avenue, 4th Floor, Boston, MA 02215, USA; [b] Harvard Medical School, Boston, MA, USA; [c] Division of Cardiology, Department of Medicine, Beth Israel Deaconess Medical Center, 185 Pilgrim Road, Palmer Building, 4th Floor, Boston, MA 02215, USA
* Corresponding author.
E-mail address: esecemsk@bidmc.harvard.edu

sensitivities and specificities for severe carotid lesions (70%–99%) with lower accuracy for moderate stenoses (50%–69%).[7]

To make a sound decision regarding referral for revascularization of patients with moderate-to-severe carotid artery stenosis, a thorough assessment of a patient's comorbidities and risk-factor profile must be made to ensure that the patient's risk of future stroke outweighs his or her risk of procedural complications. Based on current guidelines,[6,8,9] patients with severe symptomatic stenosis should be referred for carotid endarterectomy (CEA) if the perioperative risk is less than 6% (**Table 1**). Patients with moderate symptomatic stenosis have a lower risk of recurrent stroke and, thus, CEA is recommended only if the perioperative risk is less than 6%, and age, sex, and comorbidities are carefully considered.[10] For asymptomatic patients, the benefit of revascularization is more controversial because these patients have a lower risk of stroke, which makes it harder to achieve a net benefit of revascularization in this population. In addition, optimal medical therapy has improved significantly since early trials were performed (**Table 2**), potentially making it less likely to achieve a net benefit of revascularization in asymptomatic patients. In current guidelines, a perioperative risk of stroke or death less than 3% is generally recommended for asymptomatic patients being considered for revascularization (see **Table 1**).[8,9,11] Optimal medical therapy is recommended for all patients with carotid artery disease. Revascularization is not recommended for carotid lesions that are fully occluded or are less than 50% stenotic.[12]

Carotid artery stenting (CAS) and transcarotid artery revascularization (TCAR) are alternative approaches to carotid artery revascularization. More data are required to determine optimal patient selection for CEA, CAS, and TCAR. In addition, further investigation is needed to determine patient outcomes when treated with contemporary medical therapy and whether the clinical impact of this therapy should change thresholds for referral for revascularization. The use of advanced imaging techniques may refine our ability to risk-stratify patients.

EPIDEMIOLOGY AND CONSEQUENCES OF EXTRACRANIAL CAROTID ARTERY DISEASE

Approximately, 795,000 people sustain a stroke each year in the United States, and 1 of 19 deaths in the United States, in 2017, was caused by stroke. By 2030, 3.4 million additional adults older than 18 years are predicted to have suffered a stroke—a 20.5% increase in prevalence from 2012.[1] From 2014 to 2015 data, the direct medical cost of stroke in the United States was estimated to be $28 billion, and the combined direct and indirect cost was estimated to be $45.5 billion.[1]

Stroke causes significant disability and reduces the quality of life. In a survey of patient preferences, a significant proportion of patients rated major stroke as being a worse outcome than death.[13] After a stroke, patients are at risk for short-term complications including seizures, venous thromboembolism, and infection; as well as long-term complications such as pain syndromes, depression, cognitive impairment, dementia, and falls. A meta-analysis reported that approximately one-third of all stroke survivors develop depression within the first year after stroke.[14] In 2011, after hospitalization for stroke, 19% of Medicare patients required discharge to inpatient rehabilitation facilities, 25% required discharge to skilled nursing facilities, and 12% required home health care.[1]

There are significant regional, sex, and racial disparities in stroke prevalence and mortality. The median stroke prevalence in adults in the United States is 3% with the lowest prevalence in Wisconsin and the highest prevalence in Arkansas (1.9% and 4.5%, respectively). Arkansas is part of the "stroke belt," a group of states with the highest stroke mortality in the United States, which also includes North Carolina, South Carolina, Georgia Tennessee, Mississippi, Alabama, and Louisiana.[1]

Women have a higher lifetime risk of stroke than men.[1] The Framingham Heart Study identified a lifetime risk of stroke for women aged 55 to 75 years of 1 in 5 and approximately 1 in 6 for men of the same age.[15] Women have lower age-specific incidence rates of stroke than men at younger and middle ages, but similar or higher rates in older age groups. More women than men die of stroke each year due to a greater life expectancy for women. For example, women accounted for 58% of stroke deaths in 2017 in the United States.

People who are Black or Hispanic have a higher risk of stroke than White people. The age-adjusted incidence for first ischemic stroke was higher in Black (1.91/1000) and Hispanic individuals (1.49/1000) than in White individuals (0.88/1000). In 2017, non-Hispanic Black individuals had higher age-adjusted death rates from stroke than non-Hispanic (NH) White individuals.[1] Mexican Americans were found to have a higher incidence of stroke compared with NH White people (crude 3-year cumulative incidence 16.8/1000 vs 13.6/1000, respectively).

Extracranial internal carotid artery (ICA) stenosis is a major cause of ischemic stroke. It is

Table 1
Society guidelines for performing CEA in patients with symptomatic and asymptomatic carotid stenosis

	Asymptomatic	Symptomatic
2011 SVS[8]	• Consider CEA in patients with stenosis ≥60% and life expectancy >3 y with perioperative risk of stroke and death rates ≤3% (Grade I, level of evidence A)	• CEA is recommended in patients with moderate to severe carotid stenosis (50%) plus optimal medical therapy (Grade I)
2017 ESC/ESVS[9]	• Consider patients for CEA who have average surgical risk, stenosis 60%–99%, life expectancy >5 y, perioperative stroke/death rates <3%, and clinical and/or imaging characteristics associated with higher stroke risk	• Consider patients for CEA with stenosis 70%–99% if the procedural death/stroke rate is <6% (IA) • Consider patients for CEA with 50%–69% stenosis if procedural death/stroke rate is <6% (IIa)
2005 ANA[32]	• Consider for patients between the ages of 40 and 75 with stenosis 60%–99% if the patient has a 5-y life expectancy and if the surgical stroke or death frequency is <3% (Level A)	• Recommended for patients with a 5-y life expectancy and perioperative stroke/death rate <6% and 70%–99% stenosis (Level A) • Consider for patients with a 5-y life expectancy and perioperative stroke/death rate <6% and 50%–69% stenosis (Level B), but the clinician should consider additional clinical and angiographic variables (Level C)
2011 ASA/ACCF/AHA/ AANN/AANS/ACR/ ASNR/CNS/SAIP/ SCAI/SIR/SNIS/ SVM/SVS[6]	• Selection of patients should be guided by an assessment of comorbid conditions, life expectancy, and other individual factors and should include a thorough discussion of the risks and benefits of the procedure with an understanding of patient preferences (Class I, level of evidence C) • Consider in patients with >70% stenosis if the risk of perioperative stroke, MI, and death is low (IIa, level of evidence, level of evidence A)	• Recommended for patients at average or low surgical risk if the diameter of the lumen of the ipsilateral internal carotid artery is reduced more than 70% on noninvasive imaging (level of evidence A) or more than 50% in catheter angiography (level of evidence B)
2014 AHA/ASA		• CEA is recommended in patients with severe (70%–99%) stenosis if the perioperative morbidity and mortality risk is <6% (Class I, Level of evidence A) • For patients with moderate (50%–69%) stenosis, CEA is recommended depending on patient-specific factors such as age, sex, and comorbidities if the perioperative morbidity and mortality risk is <6% (Class I, Level of evidence B)

Abbreviations: AANN, American Association of Neuroscience Nurses; AANS, American Association of Neurological Surgeons; ACCF, American College of Cardiology Foundation; ACR, American College of Radiology; AHA, American Heart Association; ANA, American Academy of Neurology; ASA, American Stroke Association; ASNR, American Society of Neuroradiology; CNS, Congress of Neurological Surgeons; ESC, European Society of Cardiology; ESVS, European Society for Vascular Surgery; SAIP, Society of Atherosclerosis Imaging and Prevention; SCAI, Society for Cardiovascular Angiography and Interventions; SIR, Society of Interventional Radiology; SNIS, Society of Neuro-Interventional Surgery; SVM, Society of Vascular Medicine; SVS, Society for Vascular Surgery.

Table 2
Medical therapies used in early landmark trials compared with modern treatments

Condition	Treatment in First-Generation Trials	Modern Treatment
Antithrombotic therapy	Aspirin alone	Aspirin plus clopidogrel
Lipids	Little statin use	High-potency statins
Blood pressure	No specific target	Systolic blood pressure <130 mm Hg
Smoking cessation	No pharmacologic therapy	New pharmacologic treatments
Physical activity	No specific target	Benefits understood for regular physical activity (3 or 4 sessions of aerobic exercise per week)
Diabetes	No specific medications for CV risk	Pharmacologic treatments that reduce CV risk, hemoglobin A1C target of <7
High triglyceride levels	No specific treatment	Icosapent ethyl

Medical therapy for carotid artery stenosis has improved significantly over time.
Abbreviation: CV, cardiovascular.
From Lalla, R., Raghavan, P. & Chaturvedi, S. Trends and controversies in carotid artery stenosis treatment. *F1000Research* 9, (2020).

estimated to cause 8% to 15% of ischemic strokes or approximately 41,000 strokes per year in the United States.[3,4] In addition, TIA and stroke caused by carotid artery stenosis are associated with a high rate of recurrence of stroke.[5] Among those who have sustained an initial stroke, the risk of recurrent stroke is 25% within 5 years.[12] In ultrasound studies, the prevalence of moderate-to-severe carotid stenosis in asymptomatic patients is estimated to be 4% to 8% among adults in the United States.[16,17] The incidence of carotid stenosis increases with age. For example, in one study, severe stenosis (greater than or equal to 70%) in men ranged from 0.1% for men younger than 50 years to 3.1% (1.7%–5.3%) in men with age greater than or equal to 80 years. Similarly, among women, there was a prevalence of 0% for those less than 50 years of age and 0.9% (0.3%–1.4%) for those with age greater than or equal to 80 years.[18] Among Black individuals compared with White individuals, the risk ratio (RR) of extracranial atherosclerotic stroke was 3.18 (95% CI, 1.42–7.31) and among Hispanic individuals compared with White individuals, the RR was 1.71 (95% CI, 0.80–3.63).

PATHOPHYSIOLOGY

Cerebral ischemia caused by carotid artery stenosis may occur via several mechanisms. First, carotid atherosclerosis may develop leading to a reduction in vessel lumen diameter. Atherosclerosis most frequently occurs in the ICA. It is typically most severe at the ostium of the ICA and bifurcation of the common carotid artery and often involves the posterior wall of the artery.[19] Second, an atheroma may embolize, resulting in a distal infarct. Third, thrombus can develop on an atheroma, further narrowing the lumen of the vessel. Fourth, this thrombus may break off, leading to artery-to-artery embolic stroke. Fifth, an acute thrombotic occlusion may occur at the site of an atheroma. Sixth, a dissection of the vessel can occur.[20]

DIAGNOSIS OF CAROTID ARTERY STENOSIS

There are four primary imaging modalities used to identify carotid artery stenosis including invasive cerebral angiography, CDUS, MRA, and CTA.

Invasive cerebral angiography is the gold standard for evaluating carotid artery stenosis. The use of digital subtraction angiography reduces the dose of contrast, allows for use of smaller catheters, and provides a higher quality image of the vasculature. Advantages of this method are that it provides information about several of the head and neck arteries, and evaluates collateral flow, atherosclerotic disease in adjacent arteries, and plaque morphology and severity.[21] The primary disadvantage is that it is an invasive procedure with potential for complications. The risk of neurologic complications is approximately 1%.[22]

For this reason, noninvasive testing has essentially replaced cerebral angiography as an initial evaluation of carotid stenosis.

CDUS is recommended for the initial evaluation of a patient suspected to have carotid artery stenosis.[6] It is a noninvasive, accurate, and inexpensive method of carotid imaging. CDUS uses grayscale and Doppler ultrasound to measure the velocity of blood flow, which is translated into the severity of stenosis. The peak systolic velocity, end-diastolic velocity, spectral waveform analysis, and the ratio of the peak ICA to common carotid artery velocity (carotid index) are the standard parameters (**Fig. 1**).[23–25] More specifically, the landmark North American Symptomatic Carotid Enderterectomy Trial (NASCET) demonstrated the benefit of CEA in patients with severe carotid stenosis (greater than or equal to 70%).[12] This study used criteria designed for conventional angiography, which have now been extrapolated to CDUS. Based on NASCET criteria for CDUS, a peak systolic velocity of greater than 230 cm/s or the presence of plaque filling greater than 50% of the diameter of the vessel lumen are the primary criteria used to represent a severely stenotic lesion.[24]

CDUS has the ability to evaluate some important features of plaque morphology such as calcified and noncalcified plaques.[21] One meta-analysis reported that CDUS has a sensitivity of 89% and specificity of 84% compared with cerebral angiography for the diagnosis of a 70% to 99% lesion.[7] Importantly, the accuracy of CDUS depends on the experience of the technologist.[26] Studies may be limited by calcific lesions, patient body habitus, high carotid bifurcation, vessel tortuosity, or the presence of a carotid stent.[27] CDUS may overlook very narrow vessel lumens.[21] The presence of a complete contralateral carotid occlusion may cause overestimation of an ipsilateral carotid stenosis because of increased flow through the ipsilateral vessel.[28] New developments in CDUS technology such as contrast-enhanced ultrasound

allow for a more detailed assessment of plaque morphology but are not yet used in routine practice.[21]

MRA and CTA both provide high-resolution images of the carotid arteries. They can better determine the severity of stenosis and also provide anatomic detail of the aortic arch, which is helpful when determining treatment strategies. Advantages of MRA are that it can obtain reliable information regarding vessel stenosis in the presence of extensive arterial calcification and it does not expose patients to radiation.[21] In addition, time-of-flight (TOF)-MRA can be used in patients who are unable to receive gadolinium. One disadvantage of MRA is that it may overestimate the degree of stenosis. Both TOF-MRA and contrast-enhanced MRA are accurate for high-grade stenoses but maybe less accurate for identifying moderate stenoses.[29] CTA directly images the arterial lumen and provides an accurate assessment of vessel stenosis (see **Fig. 1**). It is particularly helpful for the identifications of complete occlusions. Significant calcification may impact the accuracy of CTA. Additional disadvantages are that iodinated contrast is generally contraindicated in patients with renal dysfunction and patients are exposed to radiation.[21]

Overall, CDUS, MRA, and CTA have high sensitivities and specificities for diagnosing carotid lesions in the 70% to 99% range with lower accuracy for stenoses in the 50% to 69% range.[7]

RISK STRATIFICATION OF PATIENTS WITH CAROTID ARTERY STENOSIS: WHO SHOULD UNDERGO REVASCULARIZATION?

Risk stratification of patients with carotid artery disease is of critical importance. The primary criteria for risk stratification include the degree of vessel stenosis, the presence of symptoms attributable to the lesion, and the comorbid conditions and operative risk of the patient. The approach to some groups, such as those with severe carotid

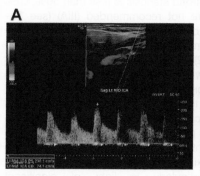
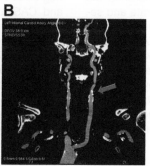

Fig. 1. Carotid duplex ultrasound and computed tomography angiography of severe stenosis in the left internal carotid artery. (*A*) Carotid duplex ultrasound doppler image of the left internal carotid artery showing a peak systolic velocity of 230.1 cm/s consistent with severe carotid artery stenosis. (*B*) Computed tomography angiography image of the same lesion revealing approximately 80% stenosis in the left internal carotid artery (*arrow*).

stenosis, symptoms attributable to the lesion, and low surgical risk, is straightforward and supported by evidence, whereas there is an ongoing debate about the management of other groups. There are several evolving strategies for risk-stratifying patients: the use of advanced imaging techniques to assess plaque morphology, the use of transcranial Doppler to detect microemboli, and the presence of silent infarcts on brain imaging.

The presence of symptoms attributable to a carotid lesion is a marker of future or recurrent stroke risk. Symptomatic disease is defined as the occurrence of focal neurologic deficits in the distribution of a carotid artery with a stenotic lesion. Nonspecific neurologic symptoms including dizziness and lightheadedness are excluded from this definition. Of note, several major clinical trials and society guidelines define symptomatic as having experienced symptoms in the last 6 months, but designated patients as asymptomatic if they had no symptoms or had experienced symptoms before 6 months.[6,30–32]

All patients, regardless of symptom status and risk-factor profile, should be treated with optimal medical therapy, which includes antiplatelet therapy, lipid-lowering therapy with an emphasis on high-intensity statins, and antihypertensive therapy (see **Table 2**).[6,8,33] Revascularization is not recommended for a complete carotid artery occlusion in any patient. Also, revascularization is not recommended for symptomatic or asymptomatic patients with mild stenosis less than 50%.[12] The risk stratification of patients with moderate and severe stenoses is more nuanced and is discussed below.

Management of symptomatic patients is more straightforward than that of asymptomatic patients as there is a clearer correlation between the degree of stenosis and the risk of stroke or stroke recurrence. Furthermore, the risk of stroke and stroke recurrence is higher in this population, so the benefits of revascularization are realized more readily. Two large, prospective, multicenter randomized control trials (RCTs) compared CEA with medical therapy alone and established the benefit of CEA in patients with moderate and severe stenotic lesions. In the NASCET trial, medical therapy alone was compared with CEA with medical therapy in symptomatic patients with different degrees of carotid stenosis.[12] All patients were treated with optimal medical therapy and were then randomized to CEA or no CEA. Optimal medical therapy included an antiplatelet agent as well as antihypertensive and lipid-lowering agents when indicated. In patients with 50% to 69% stenosis, CEA reduced the 5-year risk of death or stroke by 29%. Specifically, the 5-year risk of

ipsilateral stroke for CEA versus medical therapy alone was 15.7% versus 22.2% (RR 0.71; 95% CI 0.48–0.93; P = .045), with a number needed to treat (NNT) of 15. The risk of death or stroke at 30 days for CEA versus medical therapy was 33.2% versus 43.3% (RR 0.77; P = .005) with an NNT of 10. Subgroups that experienced the greatest benefit of CEA included men and those with recent stroke, recent hemispheric symptoms, and those taking aspirin.

In patients with greater than or equal to 70% stenosis, there was an overwhelming benefit of CEA and the trial was stopped early. When patients had been followed up for a mean of 18 months, patients who underwent CEA had a significantly lower risk of major stroke or death (8.0 vs 19.1%) and a lower risk of ipsilateral stroke (9.0 vs 26.0%). The NASCET trial excluded patients with a life expectancy less than 5 years, disabling stroke, nonatherosclerotic carotid disease, and a history of ipsilateral endarterectomy among other risk factors.

In the European Carotid Surgery Trial (ECST), 3024 patients with symptomatic carotid artery stenosis were treated with optimal medical therapy and randomized to CEA or nonoperative management. CEA was found to significantly reduce the rate of major stroke or death compared with optimal medical care alone in the subgroup of patients with greater than or equal to 80% carotid stenosis (14.9% vs 26.5%; P = .001) with NNT of 9.[31] When ECST measurement criteria were standardized to those used in NASCET, their findings were similar to those reported in NASCET.

Therefore, the current AHA/ASA guidelines recommend CEA for patients with symptomatic carotid artery stenosis in the last 6 months of severity 70% to 99% if the perioperative risk is less than 6% (Class 1A). CEA is recommended for patients with symptomatic carotid artery stenosis within the last 6 months of severity 50% to 69% if the perioperative risk is less than 6% and with consideration of patient-specific factors such age, sex, and comorbidities (Class 1B). When the degree of carotid stenosis is less than 50%, CEA and CAS are not recommended (IIIA) (see **Table 1**).[10] A better understanding of patient outcomes on modern medical therapy is needed (see **Table 2**).

Patients who have carotid artery stenosis and are asymptomatic have a lower risk of developing stroke over time compared with those who have symptomatic carotid stenosis. Therefore, the threshold to perform revascularization is higher in these patients and there is an ongoing debate about the existence of a net benefit of revascularization, particularly in light of significant improvements in medical therapy over time. Unlike patients with symptomatic carotid stenosis, the correlation between the degree of stenosis and risk of stroke is less clear for asymptomatic patients.[34] Therefore, the risks and benefits must be carefully weighed when making a recommendation for revascularization.

Early trials identified an advantage of revascularization in asymptomatic patients with carotid artery stenosis of 60% to 99%. In the Asymptomatic Carotid Atherosclerosis Study (ACAS), a prospective, RCT, 1662 patients with asymptomatic stenosis of 60% or greater were randomized to CEA or no CEA and all patients received aspirin 325 mg daily and medical risk factor management. Medical risk factor management consisted of discussions with patients regarding hypertension, diabetes, abnormal lipid levels, excessive alcohol consumption, and tobacco use. At a median follow-up of 2.7 years, the composite endpoint of ipsilateral stroke or any perioperative stroke or death was 5.1% in the CEA arm and 11.0% in the medical management alone arm (P = .004).[34] The Asymptomatic Carotid Surgery Trial (ACST-1) similarly found a significant reduction in 5- and 10-year stroke risk in asymptomatic patients younger than 75 years with carotid stenosis greater than or equal to 60%.[30] This trial reported a greater absolute risk reduction for men than for women. The ACST trial also demonstrated that the net benefit observed is delayed to approximately 2 years because of the perioperative risks (myocardial infarction and stroke). Both the ACAS and ACST trials excluded patients deemed to be at high risk for complications of CEA.

Since these trials were conducted in the 1980s and 1990s, medical therapy has evolved significantly, raising questions about whether a net benefit of revascularization still exists in asymptomatic patients with carotid artery stenosis. For example, the ACAS trial reported an annual stroke risk of 2% to 2.5% in their study cohort of patients with asymptomatic carotid stenosis of 60% to 99%.[34] In a more contemporary study published in 2007, the Second Manifestations of ARTerial disease (SMART) study reported that the risk of annual rate of stroke in asymptomatic patients with moderate to severe disease receiving optimal medical management was 1%.[35] The ongoing CREST-2 trial (ClinicalTrials.gov NCT02089217) is randomizing patients with severe, asymptomatic carotid artery stenosis to optimal medical therapy alone, CEA, or CAS and will help shed light on the role of revascularization in asymptomatic patients.[36]

Overall, the management of patients with asymptomatic carotid stenosis remains controversial and society recommendations differ (see **Table 1**). The ASA/ACCF/AHA guidelines recommend the following criteria for selection of asymptomatic patients for revascularization: (1) Patient selection should be guided by an assessment of comorbid conditions, life expectancy, and other individual factors and should include a discussion of the risks and benefits of the procedure with an understanding of patient preferences (Class I; Level of Evidence: C). (2) It is reasonable to perform CEA in asymptomatic patients who have greater than 70% stenosis if the risk of perioperative stroke, myocardial infarction (MI), and death is low (Class IIa; Level of Evidence A). (3) In patients at high risk of complications for carotid revascularization by either CEA or CAS because of comorbidities, the effectiveness of revascularization versus medical therapy alone is not well-established (Class IIb; Level of Evidence: B).[6] Given the delay in the realization of the net benefit because of perioperative adverse events in the ACAS and ASCT trials,[37] society guidelines recommend selecting patients with a life expectancy of greater than 3 to 5 years.[8,9] In the ACST trial, there was a 3.1% perioperative complication rate. Thus, the combined perioperative risk of stroke or death should be less than 3% for the surgeon and center, or risk in asymptomatic patients may exceed the overall benefit. The Society for Vascular Surgery guidelines recommend consideration of surgical intervention for patients with carotid stenosis greater than 60% if life expectancy is greater than 3 years and perioperative risk is less than 3%.[8]

Although there have not been RCTs performed to evaluate the net benefit of screening, the USPSTF recommends against routine screening for carotid disease in asymptomatic patients.[38] The 2011 ASA/ACCF/AHA guidelines recommend consideration of screening in patients with multiple cardiovascular risk factors, a carotid bruit, or those with coronary artery disease or peripheral artery disease (PAD).[6] In a study of patients with clinical evidence of arterial diseases in vascular territories other than the carotid arteries, investigators found that the prevalence of asymptomatic carotid artery disease greater than 50% was greatest in patients with PAD and abdominal aortic aneurysm.[39]

There are several areas under investigation to improve the risk stratification of patients. First, there is no definitive recommendation for the triage of asymptomatic patients with ipsilateral stroke of unknown age identified on imaging. In one prospective study, 462 patients with asymptomatic stenosis between 60% and 99% were monitored every 6 months for up to 8 years. Patients with ipsilateral stroke on their baseline CT scans had a significantly higher risk of subsequent stroke (3.6% rate of annual events vs 1.0%) at a median follow-up of 3.7 years.[40]

Second, as imaging technology evolves, noninvasive imaging techniques have been developed that can better characterize plaque morphology. Features of plaque morphology that may indicate plaque vulnerability may be used to better risk-stratify patients. MRI can identify intraplaque hemorrhage, a lipid-rich necrotic core, plaque luminal surface ulceration, and intraplaque neovascularization—features that may be associated with a higher risk of stroke.[41] CTA can identify the calcium composition of plaques. Plaques are more stable when at least 45% of their volume is made up of calcium.[41] Ultrasound can identify several features thought to increase stroke risk. These include lipid-rich plaques detected based on their echolucency and the presence of calcium, which appears as a hyperechoic plaque.[41] A newer technique of contrast-enhanced US can identify plaque neovascularization. Transcranial Doppler ultrasound can detect microemboli, which are predictive of ischemic events in both symptomatic and asymptomatic patients with carotid artery stenosis.[42] ^{18}F-fluorodeoxyglucose PET imaging, which can be paired with MRI, can identify plaque inflammation.[41] More research is needed to understand the prognostic significance of these modalities and to incorporate them into clinical care.

DETERMINING MODALITY OF REVASCULARIZATION

Once a patient has been selected to undergo revascularization, there are three primary options: CEA, CAS, and TCAR. Patient comorbidities, operative risk, life expectancy, presence of symptoms, and anatomic factors should be considered when selecting an interventional strategy.

CAS is an endovascular procedure in which a stent is placed in a carotid artery, most commonly via a transfemoral approach. Several trials have compared outcomes of CAS with CEA, including the Stenting and Angioplasty with Protection in Patients at High Risk for Endarterectomy (SAPPHIRE) trial and the Carotid Revascularization Endarterectomy versus Stent Trial (CREST). The CREST trial, a multicenter, randomized, unblinded trial, compared CAS to CEA in both symptomatic and asymptomatic patients receiving optimal medical therapy.[43] 2502 patients were randomized to either CAS or CEA. Results showed that CAS and CEA were similar in terms of the primary outcome of the composite of periprocedural stroke, MI, death, or ipsilateral stroke within 4 years of follow-up (periprocedurally: 0.7% vs 0.3%; HR 2.25; 95% CI 0.69–7.30, $P = .18$; 4-year follow-up: 10.2% vs 12.6%; HR 1.12; 95% CI 0.83–1.51; $P = .45$). In secondary analyses, the investigators found that there were more periprocedural strokes and strokes at 4 years with CAS for the

Table 3
Patient characteristics to consider when referring patients for carotid revascularization via CEA or CAS

Factor	Favors
Age >70 y	CEA
Recently symptomatic patient (<2 wk)	CEA
Tortuous and/or heavily calcified vessels	CEA
Contralateral carotid occlusion	CAS
Restenosis after prior CEA	CAS
Previous neck surgery and/or radiation	CAS
Laryngeal nerve palsy	CAS
Periprocedural risk of:	
Myocardial infarction	CAS
Cranial nerve injury	CAS
Stroke	CEA
Death	CEA
Long-term risk of:	
Myocardial infarction	No difference
Stroke	No difference
Death	No difference

From Meschia, J. F., Klaas, J. P., Brown, R. D. & Brott, T. G. Evaluation and Management of Atherosclerotic Carotid Stenosis. Mayo Clin. Proc. 92, 1144–1157 (2017).

secondary outcome of "any stroke" (periprocedurally: 4.1% vs 2.3%, P = .01; 4-year: 10.2% vs 7.9%, P = .03), but there was no difference in "major stroke" periprocedurally or at 4 years. There were fewer periprocedural MIs with CAS relative to CEA (1.1% vs 2.3%, P = .03), but no difference at 4 years. The subgroup analysis found that older patients (age greater than or equal to 70 years) had better outcomes with CEA.

The SAPPHIRE trial randomized patients at higher risk for CEA to either CEA or CAS with an embolic protection device.[44] The primary endpoint was the cumulative incidence of a composite of death, stroke, or MI within 30 days or death or stroke between days 31 and 1 year. They reported that CAS with embolic protection was not inferior to CEA in symptomatic patients with carotid artery stenosis greater than or equal to 50% or in asymptomatic patients with carotid artery stenosis of greater than or equal to 80% who had comorbid conditions that increased the risk of CEA.

Bonati and colleagues performed a meta-analysis of 16 trials (7572 patients) comparing outcomes for endovascular therapy, comprised primarily of CAS procedures, with CEA for the management of carotid artery stenosis.[45] They found that endovascular treatment was associated with an increased risk of 30-day periprocedural stroke or death compared with endarterectomy; however, in subgroup analyses, they found that this increase was only significant for patients with age greater than or equal to 70 years and there was no difference in periprocedural stroke or death for patients with age less than 70 years. Overall, patient comorbidities, anatomic features, and age must be considered when determining whether a patient should undergo CEA or CAS (**Table 3**).

TCAR is a recently developed technique for carotid artery stent placement. Access is obtained via an incision over the common carotid artery. Flow reversal is achieved which provides embolic protection. TCAR avoids potential pitfalls associated with CAS including severe PAD, challenging anatomy of the aortic arch, and a heavily calcified aorta. In a retrospective, observational study, 1182 TCAR patients were propensity matched with 10,797 CEA patients and outcomes were compared. There was no difference between TCAR and CEA in adjusted analyses of in-hospital outcomes including the combination of stroke/death/MI, stroke/death, or the individual outcomes.[46]

SUMMARY

The management and prevention of strokes caused by carotid artery disease is distinct from other causes of stroke as there is a wide range of procedural interventions available to prevent first-time stroke and stroke recurrence. In all patients, optimal medical management is of paramount importance. Patients with carotid artery stenosis must undergo a thorough assessment of life expectancy, procedural risk, comorbidities, and anatomic features to be triaged to the appropriate modality of revascularization versus optimal medical therapy alone. When revascularization is considered, further considerations are needed to determine the best revascularization strategy: CEA, CAS, or TCAR. More research is needed to understand patient outcomes on contemporary medical therapy and the optimal risk stratification of asymptomatic patients. The use of advanced imaging techniques may be able to further refine the risk stratification of these patients in the future.

CLINICS CARE POINTS

- Stroke and transient ischemic attack (TIA) caused by carotid stenosis are associated with a high rate of recurrence of stroke.

- Carotid duplex ultrasound is recommended for the initial evaluation of a patient suspected to have carotid artery stenosis.

- All patients with carotid artery disease should be treated with optimal medical therapy.

- Revascularization is not recommended for a complete carotid occlusion or patients with less than 50% stenosis.

- Patients with symptomatic stenosis of 70% to 99% should be referred for carotid endarterectomy if the perioperative risk is less than 6%.

- Patients with symptomatic stenosis of 50% to 69% have a lower risk of recurrent stroke and thus CEA is recommended for most patients if the perioperative risk is less than 6% and age, sex, and comorbidities are carefully considered.

- CEA should be considered for asymptomatic patients with carotid artery stenosis of 60% to 99% with a life expectancy greater than 3 to 5 years with perioperative risk of stroke and death less than 3%.

- When referring a patient for CEA versus carotid artery stenting or transcarotid artery revascularization, age, symptom status, and a variety of patient characteristics should be considered to triage patients to the most appropriate procedure.

- CAS may be considered for symptomatic patients with 50% to 99% stenosis with perioperative risk of less than 6% who have been deemed high risk for CEA.
- CAS may be considered for asymptomatic patients with 60% to 99% stenosis with perioperative risk of less than 3% and a life expectancy greater than 5 years who have been deemed high risk for CEA and who have clinical or imaging characteristics associated with an increased risk of stroke.

REFERENCES

1. Virani SS, Alonso A, Benjamin EJ, et al. Heart disease and stroke statistics—2020 update: a report from the American Heart association. Circulation 2020;141:e139–596.
2. Feigin VL, Forouzanfar MH, Krishnamurthi R, et al. Global and regional burden of stroke during 1990-2010: findings from the global burden of disease study 2010. Lancet 2014;383(9913):245–55.
3. Flaherty ML, Kissela B, Khoury JC, et al. Carotid artery stenosis as a cause of stroke. Neuroepidemiology 2013;40(1):36–41.
4. Hajat C, Heuschmann PU, Coshall C, et al. Incidence of aetiological subtypes of stroke in a multi-ethnic population based study: the South London Stroke Register. J Neurol Neurosurg Psychiatry 2011;82(5):527–33.
5. Marnane M, Ni Chroinin D, Callaly E, et al. Stroke recurrence within the time window recommended for carotid endarterectomy. Neurology 2011;77(8):738–43.
6. Brott TG, Halperin JL, Abbara S, et al. 2011 ASA/ACCF/AHA/AANN/AANS/ACR/ASNR/CNS/SAIP/SCAI/SIR/SNIS/SVM/SVS guideline on the management of patients with extracranial carotid and vertebral artery disease: executive summary. A report of the American College of Cardiology Foundation/American Heart Association Task Force on practice guidelines, and the American Stroke Association, American Association of Neuroscience Nurses, American Association of Neurological Surgeons, American College of Radiology, American Society of Neuroradiology, Congress of Neurological Surgeons, Society of Atherosclerosis Imaging and Prevention, Society for Cardiovascular Angiography and Interventions, Society of Interventional Radiology, Society of NeuroInterventional Surgery, Society for Vascular Medicine, and Society for Vascular Surgery. Circulation 2011;124(4):489–532.
7. Wardlaw J, Chappell F, Best J, et al. Non-invasive imaging compared with intra-arterial angiography in the diagnosis of symptomatic carotid stenosis: a meta-analysis. Lancet 2006;367(9521):1503–12.
8. Ricotta JJ, Aburahma A, Ascher E, et al. Updated Society for Vascular Surgery guidelines for management of extracranial carotid disease. J Vasc Surg 2011;54(3):e1–31.
9. Aboyans V, Ricco JB, Bartelink MEL, et al. 2017 ESC guidelines on the diagnosis and treatment of peripheral arterial diseases, in collaboration with the European society for vascular Surgery (ESVS): Document covering atherosclerotic disease of extracranial carotid and vertebral, mesenteric, renal, upper and lower extremity arteriesEndorsed by: the European stroke Organization (ESO)the Task Force for the diagnosis and treatment of peripheral arterial diseases of the European society of Cardiology (ESC) and of the European society for vascular Surgery (ESVS). Eur Heart J 2018;39:763–816.
10. Kernan WN, Ovbiagele B, Black HR, et al. Guidelines for the prevention of stroke in patients with stroke and transient ischemic attack: a guideline for healthcare professionals from the American Heart Association/American Stroke Association. Stroke 2014;45(7):2160–236.
11. Giannopoulos A, Kakkos S, Griffin MB, et al. Mortality risk stratification in patients with asymptomatic carotid stenosis. Vasc Investig Ther 2019;2:25.
12. Barnett HJ, Taylor DW, Eliasziw M, et al. Benefit of carotid endarterectomy in patients with symptomatic moderate or severe stenosis. North American Symptomatic Carotid Endarterectomy Trial Collaborators. N Engl J Med 1998;339(20):1415–25.
13. Samsa GP, Matchar DB, Goldstein L, et al. Utilities for major stroke: results from a survey of preferences among persons at increased risk for stroke. Am Heart J 1998;136(4 Pt 1):703–13.
14. Hackett ML, Pickles K. Part I: frequency of depression after stroke: an updated systematic review and meta-analysis of observational studies. Int J Stroke 2014;9(8):1017–25.
15. Seshadri S, Beiser A, Kelly-Hayes M, et al. The lifetime risk of stroke: estimates from the Framingham Study. Stroke 2006;37(2):345–50.
16. Suri MFK, Ezzeddine MA, Lakshminarayan K, et al. Validation of two different grading schemes to identify patients with asymptomatic carotid artery stenosis in general population. J Neuroimaging 2008;18(2):142–7.
17. Fine-Edelstein JS, Wolf PA, O'Leary DH, et al. Precursors of extracranial carotid atherosclerosis in the Framingham Study. Neurology 1994;44(6):1046–50.
18. de Weerd M, Greving JP, Hedblad B, et al. Prevalence of asymptomatic carotid artery stenosis in the general population: an individual participant data meta-analysis. Stroke 2010;41(6):1294–7.
19. Prasad K. Pathophysiology and medical treatment of carotid artery stenosis. Int J Angiol 2015;24(03):158–72.
20. Gonzalez NR, Liebeskind DS, Dusick JR, et al. Intracranial arterial stenoses: current viewpoints, novel

approaches, and surgical perspectives. Neurosurg Rev 2013;36(2):175.

21. Adla T, Adlova R. Multimodality imaging of carotid stenosis. Int J Angiol 2015;24:179–84.

22. Heiserman JE, Dean BL, Hodak JA, et al. Neurologic complications of cerebral angiography. AJNR Am J Neuroradiol 1994;15(8):1401–11 [discussion: 1408–11].

23. Carroll BA. Carotid sonography. Radiology 1991; 178(2):303–13.

24. Grant EG, Benson CB, Moneta GL, et al. Carotid artery stenosis: gray-scale and Doppler US diagnosis–society of Radiologists in ultrasound Consensus Conference. Radiology 2003;229(2): 340–6.

25. Huston J, James EM, Brown RD, et al. Redefined duplex ultrasonographic criteria for diagnosis of carotid artery stenosis. Mayo Clin Proc 2000;75(11): 1133–40.

26. Criswell BK, Langsfeld M, Tullis MJ, et al. Evaluating institutional variability of duplex scanning in the detection of carotid artery stenosis. Am J Surg 1998;176(6):591–7.

27. Ooi YC, Gonzalez NR. Management of extracranial carotid artery disease. Cardiol Clin 2015;33(1):1–35.

28. Fujitani RM, Mills JL, Wang LM, et al. The effect of unilateral internal carotid arterial occlusion upon contralateral duplex study: criteria for accurate interpretation. J Vasc Surg 1992;16(3):459–67 [discussion: 467–8].

29. Debrey SM, Yu H, Lynch JK, et al. Diagnostic accuracy of magnetic resonance angiography for internal carotid artery disease: a systematic review and meta-analysis. Stroke 2008;39(8):2237–48.

30. Halliday A, Harrison M, Hayter E, et al. 10-year stroke prevention after successful carotid endarterectomy for asymptomatic stenosis (ACST-1): a multicentre randomised trial. Lancet 2010;376(9746): 1074–84.

31. Randomised trial of endarterectomy for recently symptomatic carotid stenosis: final results of the MRC European Carotid Surgery Trial (ECST). Lancet 1998;351:1379–87.

32. Chaturvedi S, Bruno A, Feasby T, et al. Carotid endarterectomy–an evidence-based review: report of the Therapeutics and technology assessment subcommittee of the American Academy of Neurology. Neurology 2005;65(6):794–801.

33. Aday AW, Beckman JA. Medical management of asymptomatic carotid artery stenosis. Prog Cardiovasc Dis 2017;59(6):585–90.

34. Endarterectomy for asymptomatic carotid artery stenosis. Executive Committee for the asymptomatic carotid atherosclerosis study. JAMA 1995;273: 1421–8.

35. Goessens BM, Visseren FL, Kappelle LJ, et al. Asymptomatic carotid artery stenosis and the risk of new vascular events in patients with manifest arterial disease: the SMART study. Stroke 2007;38(5): 1470–5.

36. Available at: https://clinicaltrials.gov/ct2/show/NCT04496544. Accessed January 20, 2021.

37. Halliday A, Mansfield A, Marro J, et al. Prevention of disabling and fatal strokes by successful carotid endarterectomy in patients without recent neurological symptoms: randomised controlled trial. Lancet 2004;363(9420):1491–502.

38. LeFevre ML, U.S. Preventive Services Task Force. Screening for asymptomatic carotid artery stenosis: U.S. Preventive Services Task Force recommendation statement. Ann Intern Med 2014;161(5):356–62.

39. Goessens BM, Visseren FL, Algra A, et al. Screening for asymptomatic cardiovascular disease with noninvasive imaging in patients at high-risk and low-risk according to the European Guidelines on Cardiovascular Disease Prevention: the SMART study. J Vasc Surg 2006;43(3):525–32.

40. Kakkos SK, Sabetai M, Tegos T, et al. Silent embolic infarcts on computed tomography brain scans and risk of ipsilateral hemispheric events in patients with asymptomatic internal carotid artery stenosis. J Vasc Surg 2009;49(4):902–9.

41. Lalla R, Raghavan P, Chaturvedi S. Trends and controversies in carotid artery stenosis treatment. F1000Res 2020;9.

42. Purkayastha S, Sorond F. Transcranial Doppler ultrasound: technique and Application. Semin Neurol 2012;32(4):411–20.

43. Brott TG, Hobson RW, Howard G, et al. Stenting versus endarterectomy for treatment of carotid-artery stenosis. N Engl J Med 2010;363(1):11–23.

44. Yadav JS, Wholey MH, Kuntz RE, et al. Protected carotid-artery stenting versus endarterectomy in high-risk patients. N Engl J Med 2004;351(15): 1493–501.

45. Bonati LH, Lyrer P, Ederle J, et al. Percutaneous transluminal balloon angioplasty and stenting for carotid artery stenosis. Cochrane Database Syst Rev 2012;(9):CD000515.

46. Schermerhorn ML, Liang P, Dakour-Aridi H, et al. In-hospital outcomes of transcarotid artery revascularization and carotid endarterectomy in the Society for Vascular Surgery Vascular Quality Initiative. J Vasc Surg 2020;71(1):87–95.

Venous Thromboembolism for the Practicing Cardiologist

Abby M. Pribish, MD[a], Eric A. Secemsky, MD, MSc[b],
Alec A. Schmaier, MD, PhD[b],*

KEYWORDS

- Venous thromboembolism • Pulmonary embolism • Deep venous thrombosis • Anticoagulation
- Thrombolysis

KEY POINTS

- Venous thromboembolism is a leading cause of cardiovascular death and presents both acute and chronic challenges in patient management.
- Morbidity and mortality from pulmonary embolism are largely due to right ventricular dysfunction, and cardiologists need to be comfortable risk-stratifying and initiating therapeutic anticoagulation.
- Several advanced therapies exist to facilitate primary reperfusion. Cardiologists should be familiar with these options, including appropriate selection of patients and contraindications.
- For a majority of VTE cases, decision making regarding the duration of anticoagulation should be between time-limited treatment (3–6 months) and long-term anticoagulation.

INTRODUCTION

Venous thromboembolism (VTE), encompassing pulmonary embolism (PE) and deep vein thrombosis (DVT), is a common occurrence and can be highly morbid and fatal. In the United States alone, there are 500,000 to 600,000 PE diagnoses and 2 million DVT diagnoses annually.[1] VTE is the third leading cause of cardiovascular death in the United States.[2] Acute PE presents on a wide spectrum, from a high-risk cardiovascular emergency to an incidental finding. DVT can cause both acute and chronic vascular complications if not properly managed. The goal of this review is to ensure that cardiologists are comfortable managing VTE—including risk stratification, determining appropriate anticoagulation therapy, and assessing candidacy for advanced therapies.

PATHOPHYSIOLOGY AND NATURAL HISTORY OF VENOUS THROMBOEMBOLISM

In the late eighteenth century, Rudolf Virchow described a triad of factors which predispose to thrombosis—endothelial injury, hypercoagulability, and stasis of flow.[3] Lack of blood flow reduces expression of antithrombotic endothelial proteins within venous valves and predisposes to blood clotting.[4] Once a DVT has formed, there are several possible outcomes: fibrinolysis and spontaneous resolution, clot extension or embolization, and organization. Clot retraction happens over several days with inflammatory cell infiltration, remodeling, and eventually recanalization and reendothelialization.[5,6] Venous valves often are damaged, however, and predispose to post-thrombotic syndrome (PTS).[7]

A vast majority of PEs arise from DVTs. Acute PE may increase right ventricular (RV) afterload abruptly due to reduction in the cross-sectional area of the pulmonary arterial bed (anatomic obstruction)[8] and release of vasoconstricting agents (hypoxic vasoconstriction).[9,10] Typically, a non-preconditioned RV cannot generate a pulmonary artery pressure above 40 mm Hg.[11] RV septal bowing from pressure and volume overload leads

a Department of Medicine, Division of ADM-Housestaff, Beth Israel Deaconess Medical Center, Harvard Medical School, Deac 311, 330 Brookline Avenue, Boston, MA 02215, USA; b Division of Cardiology, Department of Medicine, Beth Israel Deaconess Medical Center, Harvard Medical School, 4th Floor, 375 Longwood Avenue, Boston, MA 02215, USA
* Corresponding author.
E-mail address: aschmaie@bidmc.harvard.edu

Cardiol Clin 39 (2021) 551–566
https://doi.org/10.1016/j.ccl.2021.06.008

to ventricular desynchrony and decreased left ventricular (LV) stroke volume, which can decrease cardiac output and lead to systemic hypotension. Supply-demand oxygen mismatch, in addition to myocyte stretch and wall stress, lead to RV ischemia and eventually obstructive shock and death—a domino-like series of events known as the "RV spiral of death."[11] Therefore, risk stratification of acute PE involves immediate assessment of hemodynamics and end-organ perfusion, focusing on the degree of RV dysfunction as the key determinate of PE severity.[11,12] The absence of hemodynamic instability does not rule out the presence of RV dysfunction, and therefore heightened PE severity.

ESTABLISHING VENOUS THROMBOEMBOLISM DIAGNOSIS

Compression ultrasound is the test of choice to establish the diagnosis of DVT, given a diagnostic accuracy of near 100% and its safety and reliability (Fig. 1). Venous Doppler waveforms should be inspected for respirophasic flow in the common femoral vein, the absence of which suggests a more proximal obstruction. CT venography or magnetic resonance venography can assess for proximal (iliac or inferior vena cava [IVC]) thrombosis or obstruction not accessible to ultrasound.[13]

CT pulmonary angiogram (CTPA) is the modality of choice to establish the diagnosis of PE, with excellent accuracy and a low rate of inconclusive studies (Fig. 2).[11,14] The ventilation/perfusion (V/Q) scan uses less radiation than CTPA and has virtually no contraindications, but results are inconclusive in approximately 50% of cases.[11,15] A pulmonary angiogram generally is considered the gold standard for definitive diagnosis but is limited in practice due to the invasive nature of the study, imaging artifacts due to incomplete respiratory maneuvers, and difficulty identifying distal, peripheral PE. Despite being a key tool in PE risk stratification, echocardiography is neither sensitive nor specific enough to establish the diagnosis of PE.[11] In cases of systemic hypotension, however, normal RV function on echocardiogram rules out PE as the cause of hemodynamic instability.

RISK-STRATIFICATION OF NEWLY DIAGNOSED VENOUS THROMBOEMBOLISM

Acute PE can be a highly morbid and fatal condition, with a mortality rate of close to 25% in hemodynamically unstable patients and still approximately 1.5% in hemodynamically stable patients.[16] PE risk stratification incorporates assessment of patient risk factors, clinical signs and hemodynamics, RV function (echo or CTPA), and cardiac biomarkers (troponin and B-type natriuretic peptide)[11] (Table 1). According to American Heart Association criteria, PE is massive if it causes a sustained drop in blood pressure greater than 40 mm Hg or a systolic blood pressure less than 90 mm Hg[17,18] and, therefore, includes PE complicated by cardiogenic shock, cardiac or respiratory arrest, or severe hypoxemia. Submassive PEs are those without hemodynamic instability but with evidence of end organ damage (such as elevated cardiac biomarkers and/or lactate) or RV dysfunction. Low risk PE has none of these features. European Society of Cardiology (ESC) criteria further subdivide submassive PE into intermediate–high risk (if both RV dysfunction and abnormal biomarkers are present) and intermediate–low risk (if either RV dysfunction or abnormal biomarkers, but not

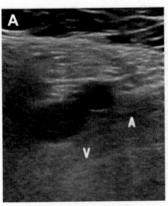
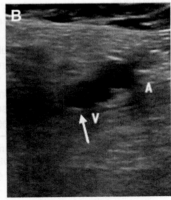
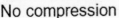

No compression   Compression

Fig. 1. Diagnosis of DVT by compression ultrasound. A 76-year-old man presented with right leg pain and swelling. Transverse B-mode ultrasound of the femoral vein without compression (A) and following compression (B) demonstrated a partially occlusive femoral vein DVT. Acute thrombus (arrow) often is echolucent and may not be apparent with visualization alone. Moderate compression should readily collapse the vein but not the artery. In the presence of DVT, the vein does not collapse (occlusive DVT) or does not collapse completely (nonocclusive DVT). A, femoral artery; V, femoral vein.

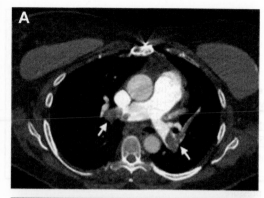

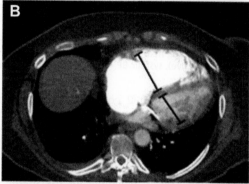

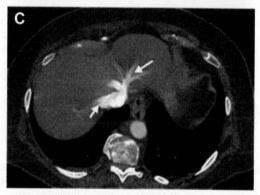

Fig. 2. Diagnosis of PE by CT pulmonary angiogram (CTPE). A 65-year-old woman presented with sudden onset dyspnea, chest pressure and lightheadedness, found to be hypotensive and hypoxemic. (*A*) Axial image demonstrated large bilateral filling defects in the main pulmonary arteries, diagnostic of PEs (*arrows*). High-risk findings present on CTPE included an enlarged RV/LV ratio greater than 1.0 on transverse 4-chamber view (*B* [*brackets*]) and IV contrast reflux into the IVC (*C* [*arrows*]).

both, are present).[11] RV dysfunction—determined by echocardiogram or by increased RV/LV ratio on CT scan—is associated with an approximately 2.5-fold increase in short-term mortality.[19,20] Some of the most common abnormalities seen on echocardiography with PE are RV enlargement, RV free wall hypokinesis, and flattening of the

interventricular septum in systole and diastole.[21] The Pulmonary Embolism Severity Index (PESI) score incorporates demographic and clinical data to predict 30-day PE mortality and can identify patients (PESI risk class I or class II) that do not require management as an inpatient.[12,22,23] Low-risk PE can generally be treated safely as an outpatient[24] and does not require a transthoracic echocardiogram (TTE) for evaluation (see **Fig. 1**).

Higher-risk DVTs tend to be more proximal in location within the venous anatomy. Acute DVT should be assessed for threatened limb, which is rare, and for risk of PTS, which is common, occurring in 20% to 50% of DVT cases with severe PTS occurring in 5%.[25] Acute high-risk DVT is characterized by phlegmasia alba (or cerulea) dolens, in which venous thrombosis is so extensive that arterial circulation is compromised. These conditions can progress to compartment syndrome and venous gangrene. Risk factors for PTS at time of DVT diagnosis include proximal (iliac or common femoral) location, preexisting venous insufficiency, obesity, and more severe VTE symptoms (eg, edema, pain, erythema) at the time of presentation (see **Fig. 2**).[7]

INITIAL ANTICOAGULATION FOR VENOUS THROMBOEMBOLISM

The initial anticoagulation management phase begins immediately upon VTE diagnosis or in cases where there is a high index of suspicion while awaiting definitive test results (**Figs. 3** and **4**). This phase lasts approximately 5 days to 21 days, and the goal is to stop active thrombosis and promote clot resolution.[26,27] Rapid systemic therapeutic anticoagulation is achieved with subcutaneous low-molecular-weight heparin (LMWH) or fondaparinux, intravenous (IV) unfractionated heparin (UFH), or the direct oral anticoagulants (DOACs) apixaban or rivaroxaban at prescribed loading doses. LMWH or fondaparinux should be preferred as the initial anticoagulant of choice in patients with VTE requiring hospitalization given their improved efficacy (perhaps in part due to a shorter time to therapeutic anticoagulation), ease of use (no requirement for drug-level monitoring or continuous IV infusion) and decreased incidence of bleeding and thrombocytopenia compared with IV UFH.[28,29] IV UFH should be reserved for cases of hemodynamic instability where advanced therapies are being considered or in patients with significant renal impairment (creatinine clearance <30 mg/dL).[11]

For outpatient treatment, DOACs are noninferior for prevention of recurrent VTE with lower bleeding risk compared with well-managed vitamin K antagonist (VKA) (eg, warfarin) therapy.[30–35]

Table 1
Pulmonary embolism severity risk stratification from European Society of Cardiology guidelines and pulmonary embolism severity index score

	Low Risk	Intermediate–Low Risk	Intermediate–High Risk	High Risk
Hemodynamic instability[a]	Absent	Absent	Absent	Present
PESI risk class[b]	<3	3–5	3–5	
RV dysfunction on TTE/CTPA	Absent	One or neither	Present	
Elevated troponin	Absent		Present	

Abbreviations: AMS, altered mental status; SBP, systolic blood pressure.

[a] Cardiac arrest, *OR* SBP less than 90 or pressors AND end organ hypoperfusion (AMS, cold/clammy, oliguria/anuria, increased lactate), *OR* persistent hypotension (SBP <90 or systolic BP drop ≥40 longer than 15 min not caused by arrhythmia, hypovolemia, or sepsis).

[b] Class 1 (score <66), class 2 (score 66–85), class 3 (score 86–105), class 4 (score 106–125), or class 5 (score >125). Score is the sum of points from each of these risk factors: +10: male, chronic lung disease, heart failure; +20: pulse greater than 110, RR ≥30, T <36C, arterial O2 sat less than 90%; +30: cancer (history or active), systolic BP <100; +60: altered mental status.

DOACs now are recommended as the first-choice anticoagulation in the acute phase for PE by multiple consensus guidelines.[11,36,37] When VKA is used in the setting of acute VTE, parenteral anticoagulation should be overlapped with VKA for at least 5 days and for 2 consecutive days upon reaching an international normalized ratio goal of 2 to 3.[11] Dabigatran and edoxaban also require initial treatment with parenteral anticoagulation for 5 days prior to initiation of oral therapy.

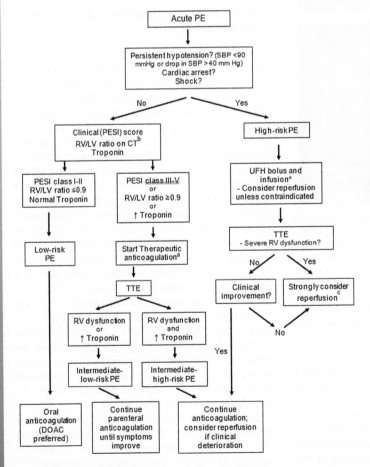

Fig. 3. Algorithm for risk stratification and management of acute PE. Management involves simultaneous assessment of clinical severity and initiation of therapeutic anticoagulation in a risk-based fashion. [a]If a patient is unable to be anticoagulated, then IVC filter placement should be considered. [b]Mild RV dilation greater than 0.9 is a frequent finding in hemodynamically stable PE. RV/LV ratio greater than or equal to 1.0 may better discriminate patients with a poor prognosis. [c]Reperfusion options include systemic or CDT or surgical or catheter-directed thrombectomy.

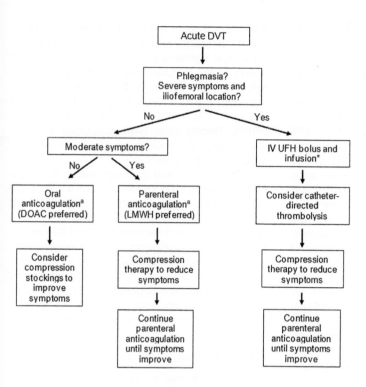

Fig. 4. Algorithm for risk stratification and treatment of acute deep venous thrombosis. Acute DVT should be assessed for signs of limb compromise and risk of PTS. [a]If a patient is unable to be anticoagulated, then IVC filter placement should be considered for proximal DVT (popliteal vein or above).

FIBRINOLYSIS AND INVASIVE VENOUS THROMBOEMBOLISM MANAGEMENT

Primary reperfusion therapies for VTE include systemic full-dose thrombolysis, systemic reduced-dose thrombolysis, catheter-directed thrombolysis (CDT) (with or without ultrasound facilitation), and mechanical thrombectomy. For patients with PE complicated by shock (systolic blood pressure <90 mm Hg) and low bleeding risk, guidelines generally recommend full-dose systemic fibrinolysis.[11,26] CDT and mechanical thrombectomy may be appropriate for patients with acute massive PE and hypotension who have moderate or high bleeding risk, failed systemic thrombolysis, or shock, which is likely to be lethal before systemic thrombolysis can take effect.[36]

Systemic Fibrinolysis

Systemic thrombolysis, typically using tissue plasminogen activator (tPA) (eg, alteplase, 100 mg, over 2 hours), carries a 3-fold risk of major bleeding over anticoagulation alone including an approximately 1% to 2% risk of intracranial hemorrhage. Systemic full-dose fibrinolysis should be reserved for massive PE only and deferred in intermediate risk PE.[38] The landmark PEITHO trial included 1005 patients with intermediate-risk PE and found that fibrinolytic therapy (tenecteplase) significantly decreased hemodynamic decompensation but increased the risk for major extracranial

bleeding and stroke, with no overall effect on mortality.[39] Following thrombolysis, anticoagulation typically is resumed when the partial thromboplastin time (PTT) is less than 1.5 times to 2 times the upper limit of normal and when fibrinogen is greater than 100 mg/dL to 150 mg/dL.

Reduced-dose systemic thrombolysis (such as tPA, 50 mg for patients 50 kg, or 0.5 mg/kg for weight <50 kg) has generated enthusiasm in management of submassive PE. Interest was based on studies performed at single centers, demonstrating similar efficacy as full-dose thrombolysis or catheter thrombolysis, with an improved safety profile.[40–42] A more recent, large retrospective study suggested, however, that half-dose thrombolysis was associated with an increased need for treatment escalation compared with full-dose thrombolysis, with no improvement in bleeding incidence.[43] Whether and how reduced-dose systemic thrombolysis should be incorporated into acute PE management currently is unclear. A large multicenter trial comparing half-dose thrombolytics to anticoagulation alone for management of intermediate-high-risk PE is under way (PEITHO-3l https://clinicaltrials.gov NCT04430569).

Catheter-directed Therapies

Facilitating local thrombolytic delivery at the site of PE in the pulmonary circulation via CDT, with or without mechanical adjunctive thrombectomy, has been a significant technical advance in PE therapy. The ideal scenario is a therapy for massive and intermediate-high risk (submassive) PE that promotes rapid hemodynamic improvement compared with standard anticoagulation, without the increased, and often unacceptable, bleeding risk of systemic thrombolysis. CDT with ultrasound-assisted low dose thrombolysis with the EKOS system (Boston Scientific, Marlborough, Massachusetts) is the most studied CDT device for treatment of submassive PE. Three small studies have demonstrated that ultrasound maceration–assisted CDT improves indices of RV function at 24 hours to 48 hours with a favorable safety profile.[44–46] In terms of clinical outcomes, however, a retrospective single-center study of 104 patients with intermediate-risk PE demonstrated that systemic anticoagulation alone resulted in similar long-term resolution of RV dysfunction, no difference in mortality, and fewer bleeding complications compared to CDT.[47] Prospective data comparing CDT to standard-of-care therapeutic anticoagulation with meaningful long-term clinical endpoints are clearly lacking.[48] A larger study comparing the EKOS device to systemic anticoagulation alone is expected to launch in 2022 (HI-PEITHO). In practice, CDT often is used with the intention of preventing hemodynamic collapse in intermediate-high-risk PE, but this indication has not yet been validated through clinical trials.[17] CDT also could be considered for use in combination with mechanical PE aspiration/maceration in the setting of massive PE or after failed systemic thrombolysis.[17]

Absolute contraindications to both locally administered and systemic thrombolytics include ischemic stroke within 3 months, prior intracranial hemorrhage, bleeding diathesis or active bleeding, structural intracranial disease, recent brain or spine surgery, or head trauma with brain injury or fracture. Relative contraindications include ischemic stroke greater than 3 months ago, current anticoagulant (eg, VKA or DOAC) use, traumatic CPR, pericarditis or pericardial effusion, pregnancy, age greater than 75 years, weight less than 60 kg, recent non-intracranial bleeding, uncontrolled hypertension (systolic blood pressure >180 mm Hg or diastolic blood pressure >110 mm Hg), recent surgery or invasive procedure, and diabetic retinopathy.[17,36]

An alternative to CDT that does not rely on thrombolysis is mechanical aspiration, which uses negative pressure to extract a more proximal pulmonary thrombus. In the FLARE study, the Flowtriever device (Inari Medical, Irvine, California) showed improvement in RV hemodynamics following mechanical thrombectomy, with a positive safety profile.[49] Similar findings were found with the Indigo Aspiration System (Penumbra, Alemeda, California) in the recently reported EXTRACT-PE trial.[50]

Surgical pulmonary embolectomy remains an option for the management of patients with high-risk PE, in particular for those presenting with massive PE and suitable surgical anatomy, clot-in-transit, intracardiac thrombi, and cardiac shunts. Recent data have supported selective use of surgical embolectomy at centers with this capability and expertise.[51]

In DVT complicated by phlegmasia, a true medical emergency, CDT should be utilized to facilitate rapid venous recanalization of the threatened limb.[36] In less-emergent DVT cases, however, it is unclear whether thrombolysis aids in the prevention of PTS compared with anticoagulation alone.[52,53] In select younger patients with iliofemoral DVT and severe symptoms, CDT should be considered. Data suggest reperfusion therapy may improve long-term quality of life through reduction in PTS severity in these patients.[54,55]

Inferior vena cava Filters

IVC filters are used as an adjunct device for the management of patients with PE and DVT. They are designed to prevent large emboli from traveling up the IVC and into the pulmonary circulation. There is no role for routine use of IVC filters. IVC filters should be considered in acute VTE only when there is a contraindication to anticoagulation or in the setting of recurrent VTE despite therapeutic anticoagulation.[36] When the contraindication has resolved and the patient is tolerating therapeutic anticoagulation, the IVC filter should be removed.[56] Despite this guideline, filter retrieval rates range from 12% to 45%.[57] IVC filters impede venous return and counter-productively serve as a nidus for venous thrombosis. Complications of IVC filters include IVC perforation, filter migration, clotting and stenosis, and PTS.[56] A meta-analysis of 11 studies, including 2 large prospective clinical trials, showed that IVC filter use decreases risk for recurrent PE but increases risk for DVT, with a nonsignificant trend toward lower PE-related mortality.[58–60] IVC filters may have more utility in patients who experience significant bleeding. A study of 1065 VTE patients who experienced major bleeding within 3 months of AC use showed that IVC filter use confers 30-day mortality benefit and a lower rate of fatal bleeding with similar risk for rebleeding or PE recurrence.[61] In patients with hemodynamically unstable PE and concomitant DVT, IVC filters often are placed to prevent a recurrent, potentially fatal PE. This strategy makes intuitive sense but data supporting this practice are limited, and it is not supported by current guidelines.[11,37,62]

WHY DID THIS PATIENT HAVE A CLOT?

Risk factors for VTE should be viewed within the entire spectrum of cardiovascular disease prevention. Age, active smoking, obesity, and hypertension are strongly associated with VTE.[63–65] There are conflicting data on the link between VTE and lipids and DM, possibly owing to publication bias or confounding by obesity, but a meta-analysis of 33 studies showed significantly higher VTE rate among patients with DM and those with dyslipidemia.[66] Statin use may aid in primary prevention of VTE.[67–69] Statins have a weak thromboprophylactic effect, thought to be due to lipid lowering, antithrombotic, and anti-inflammatory effects. Studies also have suggested that statins aid in the secondary prevention of VTE.[70,71]

Abnormalities in both exogenous and endogenous sex hormones are attributable to increased VTE risk in women. Approximately 20,000 VTE events are attributable to oral contraceptive use each year.[72,73] VTE also appears to correlate with endogenous levels of estradiol and sex hormone–binding globulin.[74]

The traditional dichotomy of provoked versus unprovoked VTE is in reality much more nuanced.[75] Provoked VTE still is associated with a significant risk of recurrence, with the exception of VTE following major trauma or surgery.[76] Perhaps what is more important is whether provoking factors are transient versus persistent.[77,78] Significant transient risk factors are any of the following within the prior 3 months: major surgery with general anesthesia for greater than 30 minutes, confined to bed in hospital greater than 3 days, fracture of lower limb, major trauma, and spinal cord injury. Minor transient risk factors are any of the following within the prior 2 months: admission to hospital for less than 3 days with acute illness, bed rest out of hospital greater than 3 days with acute illness, estrogen therapy, pregnancy or puerperium, erythropoiesis-stimulating agents, infection, IV catheters or leads, and paralytic stroke. Long-haul traveling by plane (≥8 h) is associated increased risk of VTE by approximately 3-fold compared with generation population and increases with the duration of travel.[79] The absolute risk, however, is small compared with other minor provoking factors, such as arthroscopic surgery. Persistent provoking risk factors include active cancer (not received treatment yet, treatment ongoing, or cases of treatment that is not curative), chronic inflammatory conditions especially inflammatory bowel disease, advanced age, obesity, and possibly varicose veins.

WHAT WORK-UP IS APPROPRIATE FOLLOWING UNPROVOKED VENOUS THROMBOEMBOLISM?

When evaluating the cause of unprovoked or recurrent VTE, inherited thrombophilia often is overemphasized, whereas more general cardiovascular risk factors and anatomic factors frequently are overlooked. Despite the clear heritable nature of VTE, genetic testing (such as prothrombin G20210A, factor V Leiden, or protein C, protein S or antithrombin III deficiency) is negative in the vast majority of VTE cases, and the results of testing should not be used to determine VTE management.[80] What is important is whether VTE occurred in the presence of persistent risk factors (such as inflammatory bowel disease, cancer, and obesity) or lack of a clear provoking factor. In these cases, after anticoagulation is discontinued, the risk of recurrent VTE is high (approximately 10% in first year, 16% after 2 years, 25% at 5 years, and 36% at 10 years) and is unaffected by the presence of an inherited thrombophilia.[81,82] Presence of an inherited thrombophilia should not be used to prolong treatment in a patient with clearly provoked VTE or to discontinue anticoagulation in a patient with unprovoked VTE who tests negative for a thrombophilia.[80,83,84] Furthermore, emphasis on genetics may detract from counseling on modifiable risk factors like obesity or smoking. Anatomic causes of VTE should be considered and include May-Thurner syndrome (compression of the left common iliac vein by the right common iliac artery), IVC stenosis or atresia,[85] and compression from masses or enlarged lymph nodes.

One exception to the low-yield nature of the hypercoagulable testing is identification of antiphospholipid antibody syndrome (APLAS), an autoimmune condition associated with more aggressive and recurrent thromboses in both the venous and arterial systems.[86] A diagnosis of APLAS in a patient with VTE requires positive lupus anticoagulant and/or anticardiolipin and anti–beta-2 glycoprotein 1 antibody titers at least 12 weeks apart.[80] DOACs may be less effective than VKAs at preventing VTE recurrence in APLAS.[87,88]

Data suggest that close to 10% of patients are diagnosed with cancer within a year of VTE diagnosis.[89–91] In other words, VTE may be the first clinical manifestation of cancer. Despite this, a prospective trial of limited occult-cancer screening—complete blood cell count, chest radiograph, age-appropriate screening for breast, cervical, and colon cancer—with or without comprehensive CT scan resulted in no change in the incidence of new cancer diagnosis, time to diagnosis, cancer-based mortality.[92] For a first episode of unprovoked VTE, evaluation for occult malignancy can be limited to a complete history and physical, basic laboratory testing (eg, complete blood cell count), and age-appropriate cancer screening. A more comprehensive work-up for underlying malignancy may be appropriate in patients with recurrent VTE despite anticoagulation or in patients with thrombosis at atypical locations, such as hepatic, portal, splanchnic, and cerebral veins.[93]

DURATION OF ANTICOAGULATION THERAPY AND SECONDARY PREVENTION OF VENOUS THROMBOEMBOLISM

Therapeutic anticoagulation for VTE can be divided into at least 2 phases: (1) primary treatment, where therapeutic anticoagulation actively promotes clot resolution and when risk of recurrence is highest, and, if necessary, (2) secondary prophylaxis, where the goal of anticoagulation is prevention of recurrent VTE. The primary treatment phase lasts for a minimum of 3 months, often extended to 6 months for larger clot burdens or physician preference.[37] VTE recurrence risk is elevated significantly if anticoagulation is stopped earlier than 3 months.[94,95] The goal of treatment beyond 3 months to 6 months is for secondary prevention of thrombosis. Extending anticoagulation therapy beyond 3 to 6 months reduces VTE recurrence, but, once anticoagulation is stopped, the VTE recurrence rate is the same whether the initial phase of anticoagulation was 3 months to 6 months or longer (6–18 months of additional anticoagulation).[96,97]

Recent clinical trials have established the safety and efficacy of extended anticoagulation for VTE. The AMPLIFY-EXTEND and the EINSTEIN-CHOICE trials investigated extended dosing of either full or reduced-dose apixaban (5 mg vs 2.5 mg twice daily) or rivaroxaban (20 mg vs 10 mg once daily), respectively, in patients who had already received therapeutic anticoagulation for 6 months to 12 months for VTE.[98,99] AMPLIFY-EXTEND enrolled almost exclusively patients with unprovoked VTE and compared anticoagulation to placebo whereas 60% of patients in EINSTEIN-CHOICE had a provoked VTE as their index event and the trial used low-dose aspirin as a comparator to anticoagulation. Both trials found a significant reduction in symptomatic recurrent VTE over 12 months, even with reduced-dose anticoagulation. Major bleeding rates all were less than 0.5% per year. It is important to keep in mind that low bleeding rates reflect patients who proved they already could tolerate therapeutic anticoagulation for 6 months to 12 months without significant bleeding events. These trials established extended-dosing anticoagulation as a viable option, especially in patients at high risk for VTE recurrence.[98,99]

Incorporating Bleeding Risk

The estimated risk for major bleeding while receiving anticoagulation therapy is approximately 1% to 2% over 6 months, based on prospective clinical trial data.[100,101] The RIETE and VTE-BLEED score are validated tools for stratifying bleeding risk in patients with VTE receiving anticoagulation, on the basis of variables, including history of major bleeding, age greater than or equal to 60 years, renal dysfunction, and anemia.[102,103] It is unclear how predictors of bleeding should be incorporated into decision making regarding duration of anticoagulation. None of these scoring tools has been tested in prospective trials of anticoagulation duration.[104]

To summarize, for a majority of VTE cases, decision making regarding the duration of anticoagulation should be between time-limited treatment (3–6 months) and long-term anticoagulation. In practice, it often is best to reserve decision-making regarding long-term anticoagulation until the primary treatment phase of 3 months to 6 months is completed. This time allows for patient and physician to assess tolerance of anticoagulation. Current guidelines do not recommend the use of VTE recurrence prognostic scores, D-dimer testing, or repeat imaging to determine the duration of anticoagulation. Typically, time-limited treatment is opted for provoked VTE whereas indefinite anticoagulation is usually appropriate after the first unprovoked VTE or a VTE with a chronic provoking risk factor(s).[37] One common treatment strategy is to treat patients with unprovoked VTE with 6 months of therapeutic anticoagulation, then reduced-dose anticoagulation long-term. Decisions regarding continuing anticoagulation should be reassessed at least annually, taking into account both risk of recurrent VTE and bleeding.

Aspirin for Secondary Venous Thromboembolism Prevention

Prospective clinical trials suggest that low-dose aspirin can be effective at reducing risk of recurrent VTE.[105–107] Guidelines, however, suggest using anticoagulation over aspirin for secondary prevention of VTE.[37] It is reasonable to recommend long-term aspirin therapy to patients with provoked VTE without persistent risk factors or to patients who are averse to continuing even reduced-dose anticoagulation.[36]

Combining Anticoagulation with Antiplatelet Therapy

Cardiologists are likely to care for patients with VTE who have additional indications for antiplatelet therapy. Among patients with VTE, those receiving anticoagulation plus antiplatelet therapy (either aspirin or a P2Y12 antagonist) have almost double the risk of major bleeding, with no significant impact on recurrent VTE recurrence.[108] For patients taking antiplatelet therapy for stable cardiovascular disease, guidelines recommend holding aspirin while taking anticoagulation for VTE, noting that this approach should not be applied to patients with recent acute coronary syndrome or coronary procedure.[37] Anticoagulation is as effective as antiplatelet therapy for prevention of adverse cardiovascular events[109] and only in the setting of recent stent placement is additional antiplatelet therapy likely to be indicated.

VENOUS THROMBOLISM RECURRENCE

When there is concern for recurrent VTE despite therapeutic anticoagulation, it is important to recognize that new VTE symptoms are not proof of recurrence. Incidental imaging findings suggesting presence of thrombosis must be interpreted with caution, especially in ipsilateral DVT.[110] Confirming drug compliance is essential, and then reviewing the appropriate drug choice and dosing, or underlying condition, that could lead to failure of anticoagulation.[111,112] If a patient experiences recurrent VTE despite VKA or DOAC use, then it is advised to switch to LMWH for at least 1 month, and evaluate compliance and for malignancy.[36] LMWH dosing can be increased by 1/one-fourth or one-third if recurrent VTE while on LMWH.[36,113]

SPECIAL VENOUS THROMBOEMBOLISM SCENARIOS
Cancer

Cancer and its treatment are associated with a 4-fold to-7-fold increase in risk of VTE and a higher rate of VTE recurrence.[114] Landmark studies in the pre-DOAC era established that LMWH was associated with a significant reduction in recurrent VTE compared with LMWH-bridged warfarin.[113,115,116] Parenteral options may be preferred in cases of patients intolerant of oral therapy (eg, highly emetogenic chemotherapy), but downsides of LMWH include risk of heparin-induced thrombocytopenia, and injection site reactions. Recent prospective trials comparing DOAC to LMWH for cancer patients with VTE reproduce this trend: Hokusai VTE Cancer (edoxaban),[117] SELECT-D (rivaroxaban)[118] and Caravaggio (apixaban)[119] all demonstrated noninferiority, and suggested superiority, of DOAC compared with LMWH in terms of recurrent VTE. There was a suggestion of increased bleeding, mostly gastrointestinal (GI) bleeding, especially in patients with GI malignancy and, therefore, DOACs might not be appropriate in patients with GI cancer.

Isolated Calf Deep Vein Thrombosis

Whether patients with isolated distal DVT should receive therapeutic anticoagulation is a matter of debate. The thromboembolic potential of a calf vein DVT is low,[120] and, in low-risk patients, the 3-month thromboembolic risk is similar whether or not patients with isolated distal DVT receive anticoagulation.[121] Therefore, deferring AC could be reasonable in the absence of risk factors such as history of prior VTE, active malignancy, or inpatient status.[122] Follow-up ultrasound(s) can be effective for surveillance, with anticoagulation reserved for cases of clot extension. In the OPTIMEV study, isolated distal DVT was associated a similar risk of death, major bleeding, and rate of VTE recurrence compared with those proximal VTE.[123] Furthermore, if a patient is low-risk but symptomatic, it often is practical to treat isolated calf DVT with a 3-month course of anticoagulation to improve symptoms and decrease risk of PTS.[36,124]

Subsegmental pulmonary embolism

In patients with subsegmental PE and no proximal DVT, guidelines favor clinical surveillance over anticoagulation, if a patient is low risk for recurrent VTE, namely no immobilization or hospitalized status, malignancy, or other provoking factor.[36] This applies mostly to incidentally detected PE.[125] One also should make every effort to confirm that the subsegmental diagnosis is a true positive.[36] In patients with symptoms that can be attributed to the subsegmental PE, it is reasonable to treat with a course of anticoagulation for 3 months, assuming the patient is at low risk for bleeding. There is poor correlation between clot location (proximal vs distal) and PE symptom burden. Clinical trials testing whether anticoagulation can be withheld safely in isolated subsegmental PE currently are under way (SAFE-SSPE and STOPAPE; https://clinicaltrials.gov NCT04263038 and NCT04727437, respectively).

Catheter-associated Thrombosis

Between 50% and 90% of upper extremity DVTs are associated with a central venous line (CVL).[126] Patients with a CVL-associated DVT should receive anticoagulation for 3 months or until the CVL is removed, whichever is longer.[127] If the CVL is functional (can flush and infuse), the line does not have to be removed and is safe to use in presence of a thrombus.[26,127] Anticoagulation alone should reduce symptoms (ie, swelling and limb pain) associated with catheter-related thrombosis. If the line is not functional or no longer required, it should be removed, becuases this facilitate thrombus resolution. The optimal time between initiation of anticoagulation and removal of the CVL has not been established but in general, once therapeutic anticoagulation has been administered for 24 hours to 72 hours, it is reasonable to remove the catheter.

Obesity

The International Society on Thrombosis and Haemostasis 2016 guidelines discouraged use of DOACs for morbidly obese patients (body mass index >40 kg/m^2, weight >120 kg), unless drug-specific peak/trough levels could be obtained (eg, anti–factor Xa for apixaban, rivaroxaban, or edoxaban).[128] These tests often are not available in standard clinical laboratories. Pharmacokinetic data on DOAC levels and efficacy in obesity are limited.[129] In a study of 1840 obese (weight >100 kg and <300 kg) patients with acute VTE, there was no difference in rate of VTE recurrence or bleeding within 1 year between patients receiving DOACs and warfarin.[130] Nevertheless, the authors recommend caution using DOACs for the primary treatment phase of VTE in patients with morbid obesity.

Bariatric surgery can have an impact on medication absorption and metabolism given postsurgical changes to the transit time, surface area, pH, and blood flow of the GI tract. Given that these changes are variable with difficult to predict impact on medication absorption, which has not been extensively studied for DOACs, warfarin typically is recommended over a DOAC in the bariatric surgery population.[131]

POST–VENOUS THROMBOEMBOLISM COMPLICATIONS

Post-PE syndrome involves functional impairment, quality of life reduction, dyspnea, or exercise intolerance, which are attributable to the long-term impact of PE on pulmonary gas exchange, pulmonary arterial flow dynamics, and cardiac function. There are no guideline recommended treatments for post-PE syndrome.[132] Chronic thromboembolic pulmonary hypertension (CTEPH) is another feared complication of PE. The rate of CTEPH development after acute PE is thought to be 0.4% to 9.1%; routine screening for CTEPH is not recommended after acute PE and V/Q is the preferred imaging modality to evaluate for CTEPH.[133]

PTS occurs in as many as 50% of patients following DVT and includes leg heaviness, fatigue, or swelling (mild/moderate forms) or severe pain, chronic ulceration, and refractory edema (severe form).[134,135] Undertreatment or delayed initiation of anticoagulation following DVT is a major risk factor. Compression therapy, 20 mm Hg to 30 mm Hg usually, is appropriate for patients with PTS, especially if there is edema.[7,36] Venous ulcer management requires wound care management, including compression, leg elevation, and regular dressing changes with a dedicated wound care specialist. Treatment options for PTS are limited and prevention remains the best management. Unfortunately, data do not support routine use of compression stockings to prevent PTS following DVT.[136] Compression of 20 mm Hg to 30 mm Hg (or as much as tolerated), however, can reduce the swelling and pain of acute DVT. Patients with these symptoms are at higher risk to develop PTS.[7] It often is not possible to obtain fitted compression stockings a the hospital—in the acute setting, leg wrapping is appropriate. Compression therapy is safe during acute DVT. There is no evidence that embolism risk increased in those with DVT who have compression stockings.

SUMMARY

Practicing cardiologists should be comfortable managing VTE. DOACs have emerged as the preferred first-line anticoagulation strategy in a majority of VTE scenarios. Use of novel technologies, such as CDT and suction thrombectomy, are expanding, yet prospective trials are required to establish whether aggressive upfront reperfusion using catheter therapies or low-dose thrombolysis improves outcomes in intermediate-high-risk PE. Large randomized clinical trials have established the safety and efficacy of extended anticoagulation therapy with DOACs for secondary prevention of VTE. VTE risk factors overlap considerably with standard cardiovascular disease risk factors, and VTE prevention should be in mind when cardiologists discuss lifestyle modifications and medical optimization with their patients.

CLINICS CARE POINTS

- Early risk-stratification and initiation of therapeutic anticoagulation is critical in management of VTE.

- Outside of massive PE, there is no routine role for advanced therapies (fibrinolysis, catheter-directed therapies, etc.).

- Duration of anticoagulation for VTE should typically be either be time-limited (3-6 months) for provoked VTE or indefinite for unprovoked VTE.

DISCLOSURE

EAS has the following disclosures: speaking and consultation fees from Abbott, Bayer, Beckton Dickinson, Boston Scientific, Cook, Cardiovascular Systems Inc., Inari, Janssen, Medtronic, Philips, and VentureMed. The other authors have nothing to disclose.

ACKNOWLEDGMENTS

EAS is supported by NIH K23-HL150290, a Miles Shore Faculty Development Award from Harvard Medical School and research support from Astra-Zeneca, Beckton Dickinson, Boston Scientific, Cook, Cardiovascular Systems Inc., Laminate Medical, Medtronic and Philips. AAS is supported by a Mentored Research Award from the Thrombosis and Hemostasis Research Society, research funding from the North American Thrombosis Forum, and by the John S. LaDue Memorial Fellowship from Harvard Medical School.

REFERENCES

1. Giordano NJ, Jansson PS, Young MN, et al. Epidemiology, pathophysiology, stratification, and natural history of pulmonary embolism. Tech Vasc Interv Radiol 2017;20(3):135–40.
2. Goldhaber SZ, Bounameaux H. Pulmonary embolism and deep vein thrombosis. Lancet 2012; 379(9828):1835–46.
3. Virchow R. Gesammelte Abhandlungen zur Wissenschaftlichen Medicin. Frankfurt (Germany): Meidinger Sohn & Comp; 1856.
4. Welsh JD, Hoofnagle MH, Bamezai S, et al. Hemodynamic regulation of perivalvular endothelial gene expression prevents deep venous thrombosis. J Clin Invest 2019;129(12):5489–500.
5. Kearon C. Natural history of venous thromboembolism. Circulation 2003;107(23 Suppl 1):I22–30.
6. Markel A. Origin and natural history of deep vein thrombosis of the legs. Semin Vasc Med 2005; 5(1):65–74.
7. Rabinovich A, Kahn SR. How I treat the postthrombotic syndrome. Blood 2018;131(20):2215–22.
8. McIntyre KM, Sasahara AA. The hemodynamic response to pulmonary embolism in patients without prior cardiopulmonary disease. Am J Cardiol 1971;28(3):288–94.
9. Smulders YM. Pathophysiology and treatment of haemodynamic instability in acute pulmonary embolism: the pivotal role of pulmonary vasoconstriction. Cardiovasc Res 2000;48(1):23–33.
10. Burrowes KS, Clark AR, Tawhai MH. Blood flow redistribution and ventilation-perfusion mismatch during embolic pulmonary arterial occlusion. Pulm Circ 2011;1(3):365–76.
11. Konstantinides SV, Meyer G, Becattini C, et al. 2019 ESC guidelines for the diagnosis and management of acute pulmonary embolism developed in collaboration with the European Respiratory Society (ERS): the task force for the diagnosis and management of acute pulmonary embolism of the European Society of Cardiology (ESC). Eur Respir J 2019;54(3). https://doi.org/10.1183/13993003. 01647-2019.
12. Lankeit M, Jiménez D, Kostrubiec M, et al. Predictive value of the high-sensitivity troponin T assay and the simplified Pulmonary Embolism Severity Index in hemodynamically stable patients with acute pulmonary embolism: a prospective validation study. Circulation 2011;124(24):2716–24.
13. Katz DS, Fruauff K, Kranz A-O, et al. Imaging of deep venous thrombosis: a multimodality overview. Appl Radiol 2014;43:6–16.
14. Stein PD, Fowler SE, Goodman LR, et al. Multidetector computed tomography for acute pulmonary embolism. N Engl J Med 2006;354(22):2317–27.
15. Sostman HD, Coleman RE, DeLong DM, et al. Evaluation of revised criteria for ventilation-perfusion scintigraphy in patients with suspected pulmonary embolism. Radiology 1994;193(1):103–7.
16. Casazza F, Becattini C, Bongarzoni A, et al. Clinical features and short term outcomes of patients with acute pulmonary embolism. The Italian Pulmonary Embolism Registry (IPER). Thromb Res 2012; 130(6):847–52.
17. Giri J, Sista AK, Weinberg I, et al. Interventional therapies for acute pulmonary embolism: current status and principles for the development of novel evidence: a scientific statement from the American Heart Association. Circulation 2019;140(20): e774–801.
18. Jaff MR, McMurtry MS, Archer SL, et al. Management of massive and submassive pulmonary embolism, iliofemoral deep vein thrombosis, and chronic thromboembolic pulmonary hypertension:

a scientific statement from the American Heart Association. Circulation 2011;123(16):1788–830.

19. Cho JH, Kutti Sridharan G, Kim SH, et al. Right ventricular dysfunction as an echocardiographic prognostic factor in hemodynamically stable patients with acute pulmonary embolism: a meta-analysis. BMC Cardiovasc Disord 2014;14:64.

20. Meinel FG, Nance JW Jr, Schoepf UJ, et al. Predictive value of computed tomography in acute pulmonary embolism: systematic review and meta-analysis. Am J Med 2015;128(7):747–59.e2.

21. Kurnicka K, Lichodziejewska B, Goliszek S, et al. Echocardiographic pattern of acute pulmonary embolism: analysis of 511 consecutive patients. J Am Soc Echocardiogr 2016;29(9):907–13.

22. Aujesky D, Roy PM, Verschuren F, et al. Outpatient versus inpatient treatment for patients with acute pulmonary embolism: an international, open-label, randomised, non-inferiority trial. Lancet 2011; 378(9785):41–8.

23. Aujesky D, Obrosky DS, Stone RA, et al. Derivation and validation of a prognostic model for pulmonary embolism. Am J Respir Crit Care Med 2005;172(8): 1041–6.

24. Islam EA, Winn RE, Test V. Management of low-risk pulmonary embolism. Clin Chest Med 2018;39(3): 561–8.

25. Prandoni P, Kahn SR. Post-thrombotic syndrome: prevalence, prognostication and need for progress. Br J Haematol 2009;145(3):286–95.

26. Lyman GH, Carrier M, Ay C, et al. American Society of Hematology 2021 guidelines for management of venous thromboembolism: prevention and treatment in patients with cancer. Blood Adv 2021; 5(4):927–74.

27. Renner E, Barnes GD. Antithrombotic management of venous thromboembolism: JACC focus seminar. J Am Coll Cardiol 2020;76(18):2142–54.

28. Erkens PM, Prins MH. Fixed dose subcutaneous low molecular weight heparins versus adjusted dose unfractionated heparin for venous thromboembolism. Cochrane Database Syst Rev 2010;(9): CD001100.

29. Stein PD, Hull RD, Matta F, et al. Incidence of thrombocytopenia in hospitalized patients with venous thromboembolism. Am J Med 2009;122(10):919–30.

30. Chan NC, Eikelboom JW, Weitz JI. Evolving treatments for arterial and venous thrombosis: role of the direct oral anticoagulants. Circ Res 2016; 118(9):1409–24.

31. Becattini C, Agnelli G. Treatment of venous thromboembolism with new anticoagulant agents. J Am Coll Cardiol 2016;67(16):1941–55.

32. Schulman S, Kearon C, Kakkar AK, et al. Dabigatran versus warfarin in the treatment of acute venous thromboembolism. N Engl J Med 2009; 361(24):2342–52.

33. Bauersachs R, Berkowitz SD, Brenner B, et al. Oral rivaroxaban for symptomatic venous thromboembolism. N Engl J Med 2010;363(26):2499–510.

34. Büller HR, Prins MH, Lensin AW, et al. Oral rivaroxaban for the treatment of symptomatic pulmonary embolism. N Engl J Med 2012;366(14):1287–97.

35. Agnelli G, Buller HR, Cohen A, et al. Oral apixaban for the treatment of acute venous thromboembolism. N Engl J Med 2013;369(9):799–808.

36. Kearon C, Akl EA, Ornelas J, et al. Antithrombotic therapy for VTE disease: CHEST guideline and expert panel report. Chest 2016;149(2):315–52.

37. Ortel TL, Neumann I, Ageno W, et al. American Society of Hematology 2020 guidelines for management of venous thromboembolism: treatment of deep vein thrombosis and pulmonary embolism. Blood Adv 2020;4(19):4693–738.

38. Marti C, John G, Konstantinides S, et al. Systemic thrombolytic therapy for acute pulmonary embolism: a systematic review and meta-analysis. Eur Heart J 2015;36(10):605–14.

39. Meyer G, Vicaut E, Danays T, et al. Fibrinolysis for patients with intermediate-risk pulmonary embolism. N Engl J Med 2014;370(15):1402–11.

40. Sharifi M, Bay C, Skrocki L, et al. Moderate pulmonary embolism treated with thrombolysis (from the "MOPETT" trial). Am J Cardiol 2013;111(2):273–7.

41. Sharifi M, Awdisho A, Schroeder B, et al. Retrospective comparison of ultrasound facilitated catheter-directed thrombolysis and systemically administered half-dose thrombolysis in treatment of pulmonary embolism. Vasc Med 2019;24(2):103–9.

42. Wang C, Zhai Z, Yang Y, et al. Efficacy and safety of low dose recombinant tissue-type plasminogen activator for the treatment of acute pulmonary thromboembolism: a randomized, multicenter, controlled trial. Chest 2010;137(2):254–62.

43. Kiser TH, Burnham EL, Clark B, et al. Half-dose versus full-dose alteplase for treatment of pulmonary embolism. Crit Care Med 2018;46(10): 1617–25.

44. Kucher N, Boekstegers P, Müller OJ, et al. Randomized, controlled trial of ultrasound-assisted catheter-directed thrombolysis for acute intermediate-risk pulmonary embolism. Circulation 2014;129(4):479–86.

45. Piazza G, Hohlfelder B, Jaff MR, et al. A prospective, single-arm, multicenter trial of ultrasound-facilitated, catheter-directed, low-dose fibrinolysis for acute massive and submassive pulmonary embolism: the SEATTLE II study. JACC Cardiovasc Interv 2015;8(10):1382–92.

46. Tapson VF, Sterling K, Jones N, et al. A randomized trial of the optimum duration of acoustic pulse thrombolysis procedure in acute intermediate-risk pulmonary embolism: the OPTALYSE PE trial. JACC Cardiovasc Interv 2018;11(14):1401–10.

47. Schissler AJ, Gylnn RJ, Sobieszczyk PS, et al. Ultrasound-assisted catheter-directed thrombolysis compared with anticoagulation alone for treatment of intermediate-risk pulmonary embolism. Pulm Circ 2018;8(4). 2045894018800265.

48. Konstantinides SV, Barco S. Prevention of early complications and late consequences after acute pulmonary embolism: focus on reperfusion techniques. Thromb Res 2018;164:163–9.

49. Tu T, Toma C, Tapson VF, et al. A prospective, single-arm, multicenter trial of catheter-directed mechanical thrombectomy for intermediate-risk acute pulmonary embolism: the FLARE study. JACC Cardiovasc Interv 2019;12(9):859–69.

50. Janssen EM, Dy SM, Meara AS, et al. Analysis of patient preferences in lung cancer - estimating acceptable tradeoffs between treatment benefit and side effects. Patient Prefer Adherence 2020; 14:927–37.

51. Goldberg JB, Spevack DM, Ahsan S, et al. Survival and right ventricular function after surgical management of acute pulmonary embolism. J Am Coll Cardiol 2020;76(8):903–11.

52. Enden T, Haig Y, Kløw NE, et al. Long-term outcome after additional catheter-directed thrombolysis versus standard treatment for acute iliofemoral deep vein thrombosis (the CaVenT study): a randomised controlled trial. Lancet 2012; 379(9810):31–8.

53. Vedantham S, Goldhaber SZ, Julian JA, et al. Pharmacomechanical catheter-directed thrombolysis for deep-vein thrombosis. N Engl J Med 2017; 377(23):2240–52.

54. Kahn SR, Julian JA, Kearon C, et al. Quality of life after pharmacomechanical catheter-directed thrombolysis for proximal deep venous thrombosis. J Vasc Surg Venous Lymphat Disord 2020;8(1): 8–23.e18.

55. Nathan AS, Giri J. Reexamining the open-vein hypothesis for acute deep venous thrombosis. Circulation 2019;139(9):1174–6.

56. Duffett L, Carrier M. Inferior vena cava filters. J Thromb Haemost 2017;15(1):3–12.

57. Angel LF, Tapson V, Galgon RE, et al. Systematic review of the use of retrievable inferior vena cava filters. J Vasc Interv Radiol 2011;22(11): 1522–30.e3.

58. Bikdeli B, Chatterjee S, Desai NR, et al. Inferior vena cava filters to prevent pulmonary embolism: systematic review and meta-analysis. J Am Coll Cardiol 2017;70(13):1587–97.

59. Decousus H, Leizorovicz A, Parent F, et al. A clinical trial of vena caval filters in the prevention of pulmonary embolism in patients with proximal deep-vein thrombosis. Prévention du Risque d'Embolie Pulmonaire par Interruption Cave Study Group. N Engl J Med 1998;338(7):409–15.

60. Mismetti P, Laporte S, Pellerin O, et al. Effect of a retrievable inferior vena cava filter plus anticoagulation vs anticoagulation alone on risk of recurrent pulmonary embolism: a randomized clinical trial. JAMA 2015;313(16):1627–35.

61. Mellado M, Trujillo-Santos J, Bikdeli B, et al. Vena cava filters in patients presenting with major bleeding during anticoagulation for venous thromboembolism. Intern Emerg Med 2019;14(7):1101–12.

62. Stein PD, Matta F, Keyes DC, et al. Impact of vena cava filters on in-hospital case fatality rate from pulmonary embolism. Am J Med 2012;125(5):478–84.

63. Wattanakit K, Lutsey PL, Bell EJ, et al. Association between cardiovascular disease risk factors and occurrence of venous thromboembolism. A time-dependent analysis. Thromb Haemost 2012; 108(3):508–15.

64. Gregson J, Kaptoge S, Bolton T, et al. Cardiovascular risk factors associated with venous thromboembolism. JAMA Cardiol 2019;4(2):163–73.

65. Cushman M. Epidemiology and risk factors for venous thrombosis. Semin Hematol 2007;44(2): 62–9.

66. Mi Y, Yan S, Lu Y, et al. Venous thromboembolism has the same risk factors as atherosclerosis: a PRISMA-compliant systemic review and meta-analysis. Medicine (Baltimore) 2016;95(32):e4495.

67. Skajaa N, Szépligeti SK, Horváth-Puhó E, et al. Initiation of statins and risk of venous thromboembolism: population-based matched cohort study. Thromb Res 2019;184:99–104.

68. Kunutsor SK, Seidu S, Khunti K. Statins and primary prevention of venous thromboembolism: a systematic review and meta-analysis. Lancet Haematol 2017;4(2):e83–93.

69. Glynn RJ, Danielson E, Fonseca FA, et al. A randomized trial of rosuvastatin in the prevention of venous thromboembolism. N Engl J Med 2009; 360(18):1851–61.

70. Biere-Rafi S, Hutten BA, Squizzato A, et al. Statin treatment and the risk of recurrent pulmonary embolism. Eur Heart J 2013;34(24):1800–6.

71. Kunutsor SK, Seidu S, Khunti K. Statins and secondary prevention of venous thromboembolism: pooled analysis of published observational cohort studies. Eur Heart J 2017;38(20):1608–12.

72. Tchaikovski SN, Rosing J. Mechanisms of estrogen-induced venous thromboembolism. Thromb Res 2010;126(1):5–11.

73. Eischer L, Eichinger S, Kyrle PA. The risk of recurrence in women with venous thromboembolism while using estrogens: a prospective cohort study. J Thromb Haemost 2014;12(5):635–40.

74. Scheres LJJ, van Hylckama Vlieg A, Ballieux B, et al. Endogenous sex hormones and risk of venous thromboembolism in young women. J Thromb Haemost 2019;17(8):1297–304.

75. Albertsen IE, Piazza G, Goldhaber SZ. Let's stop dichotomizing venous thromboembolism as provoked or unprovoked. Circulation 2018;138(23):2591–3.

76. Albertsen IE, Nielsen PB, Søgaard M, et al. Risk of recurrent venous thromboembolism: a Danish Nationwide cohort study. Am J Med 2018;131(9): 1067–74.e4.

77. Anderson FA Jr, Spencer FA. Risk factors for venous thromboembolism. Circulation 2003; 107(23 Suppl 1):I9–16.

78. Rogers MA, Levine DA, Blumberg N, et al. Triggers of hospitalization for venous thromboembolism. Circulation 2012;125(17):2092–9.

79. Chandra D, Parisini E, Mozaffarian D. Meta-analysis: travel and risk for venous thromboembolism. Ann Intern Med 2009;151(3):180–90.

80. Connors JM. Thrombophilia testing and venous thrombosis. N Engl J Med 2017;377(12):1177–87.

81. Khan F, Rahman A, Carrier M, et al. Long term risk of symptomatic recurrent venous thromboembolism after discontinuation of anticoagulant treatment for first unprovoked venous thromboembolism event: systematic review and meta-analysis. BMJ 2019;366: l4363.

82. Baglin T, Luddington R, Brown K, et al. Incidence of recurrent venous thromboembolism in relation to clinical and thrombophilic risk factors: prospective cohort study. Lancet 2003;362(9383):523–6.

83. Stern RM, Al-Samkari H, Connors JM. Thrombophilia evaluation in pulmonary embolism. Curr Opin Cardiol 2019;34(6):603–9.

84. Stevens SM, Ansell JE. Thrombophilic evaluation in patients with acute pulmonary embolism. Semin Respir Crit Care Med 2017;38(1):107–20.

85. Shi W, Dowell JD. Etiology and treatment of acute inferior vena cava thrombosis. Thromb Res 2017; 149:9–16.

86. Garcia D, Akl EA, Carr R, et al. Antiphospholipid antibodies and the risk of recurrence after a first episode of venous thromboembolism: a systematic review. Blood 2013;122(5):817–24.

87. Malec K, Broniatowska E, Undas A. Direct oral anticoagulants in patients with antiphospholipid syndrome: a cohort study. Lupus 2020;29(1): 37–44.

88. Pengo V, Denas G, Zoppellaro G, et al. Rivaroxaban vs warfarin in high-risk patients with antiphospholipid syndrome. Blood 2018;132(13):1365–71.

89. Carrier M, Le Gal G, Wells PS, et al. Systematic review: the Trousseau syndrome revisited: should we screen extensively for cancer in patients with venous thromboembolism? Ann Intern Med 2008; 149(5):323–33.

90. White RH, Chew HK, Zhou H, et al. Incidence of venous thromboembolism in the year before the diagnosis of cancer in 528,693 adults. Arch Intern Med 2005;165(15):1782–7.

91. Sørensen HT, Mellemkjaer L, Steffensen FH, et al. The risk of a diagnosis of cancer after primary deep venous thrombosis or pulmonary embolism. N Engl J Med 1998;338(17):1169–73.

92. Carrier M, Lazo-Langner A, Shivakumar S, et al. Screening for occult cancer in unprovoked venous thromboembolism. N Engl J Med 2015;373(8): 697–704.

93. Jara-Palomares L, Otero R, Jimenez D, et al. Development of a risk prediction score for occult cancer in patients with VTE. Chest 2017;151(3): 564–71.

94. Kearon C, Akl EA. Duration of anticoagulant therapy for deep vein thrombosis and pulmonary embolism. Blood 2014;123(12):1794–801.

95. Boutitie F, Pinede L, Schulman S, et al. Influence of preceding length of anticoagulant treatment and initial presentation of venous thromboembolism on risk of recurrence after stopping treatment: analysis of individual participants' data from seven trials. BMJ 2011;342:d3036.

96. Couturaud F, Sanchez O, Pernod G, et al. Six months vs extended oral anticoagulation after a first episode of pulmonary embolism: the PADIS-PE randomized clinical trial. JAMA 2015;314(1):31–40.

97. Schulman S, Kearon C, Kakkar AK, et al. Extended use of dabigatran, warfarin, or placebo in venous thromboembolism. N Engl J Med 2013;368(8): 709–18.

98. Agnelli G, Buller HR, Cohen A, et al. Apixaban for extended treatment of venous thromboembolism. N Engl J Med 2013;368(8):699–708.

99. Weitz JI, Lensing AWA, Prins MH, et al. Rivaroxaban or aspirin for extended treatment of venous thromboembolism. N Engl J Med 2017;376(13): 1211–22.

100. van Es N, Coppens M, Schulman S, et al. Direct oral anticoagulants compared with vitamin K antagonists for acute venous thromboembolism: evidence from phase 3 trials. Blood 2014;124(12): 1968–75.

101. Carrier M, Le Gal G, Wells PS, et al. Systematic review: case-fatality rates of recurrent venous thromboembolism and major bleeding events among patients treated for venous thromboembolism. Ann Intern Med 2010;152(9):578–89.

102. Nishimoto Y, Yamashita Y, Morimoto T, et al. Validation of the VTE-BLEED score's long-term performance for major bleeding in patients with venous thromboembolisms: from the COMMAND VTE registry. J Thromb Haemost 2020;18(3): 624–32.

103. Ruíz-Giménez N, Suárez C, González R, et al. Predictive variables for major bleeding events in patients presenting with documented acute venous thromboembolism. Findings from the RIETE registry. Thromb Haemost 2008;100(1):26–31.

104. Klok FA, Huisman MV. How I assess and manage the risk of bleeding in patients treated for venous thromboembolism. Blood 2020;135(10):724–34.

105. Becattini C, Agnelli G, Schenone A, et al. Aspirin for preventing the recurrence of venous thromboembolism. N Engl J Med 2012;366(21): 1959–67.

106. Brighton TA, Eikelboom JW, Mann K, et al. Low-dose aspirin for preventing recurrent venous thromboembolism. N Engl J Med 2012;367(21):1979–87.

107. Simes J, Becattini C, Agnelli G, et al. Aspirin for the prevention of recurrent venous thromboembolism: the INSPIRE collaboration. Circulation 2014; 130(13):1062–71.

108. Valeriani E, Porreca E, Weitz JI, et al. Impact of concomitant antiplatelet therapy on the efficacy and safety of direct oral anticoagulants for acute venous thromboembolism: systematic review and meta-analysis. J Thromb Haemost 2020;18(7): 1661–71.

109. Hurlen M, Abdelnoor M, Smith P, et al. Warfarin, aspirin, or both after myocardial infarction. N Engl J Med 2002;347(13):969–74.

110. Barco S, Konstantinides S, Huisman MV, et al. Diagnosis of recurrent venous thromboembolism. Thromb Res 2018;163:229–35.

111. Schulman S. How I treat recurrent venous thromboembolism in patients receiving anticoagulant therapy. Blood 2017;129(25):3285–93.

112. Kyrle PA. How I treat recurrent deep-vein thrombosis. Blood 2016;127(6):696–702.

113. Lee AY, Levine MN, Baker RI, et al. Low-molecular-weight heparin versus a coumarin for the prevention of recurrent venous thromboembolism in patients with cancer. N Engl J Med 2003;349(2): 146–53.

114. Blom JW, Doggen CJ, Osanto S, et al. Malignancies, prothrombotic mutations, and the risk of venous thrombosis. JAMA 2005;293(6): 715–22.

115. Lee AYY, Kamphuisen PW, Meyer G, et al. Tinzaparin vs warfarin for treatment of acute venous thromboembolism in patients with active cancer: a randomized clinical trial. JAMA 2015;314(7): 677–86.

116. Posch F, Königsbrügge O, Zielinski C, et al. Treatment of venous thromboembolism in patients with cancer: a network meta-analysis comparing efficacy and safety of anticoagulants. Thromb Res 2015;136(3):582–9.

117. Raskob GE, van Es N, Verhamme P, et al. Edoxaban for the treatment of cancer-associated venous thromboembolism. N Engl J Med 2018;378(7): 615–24.

118. Young AM, Marshall A, Thirlwall J, et al. Comparison of an oral factor Xa inhibitor with low molecular weight heparin in patients with cancer with venous thromboembolism: results of a randomized trial (SELECT-D). J Clin Oncol 2018;36(20): 2017–23.

119. Agnelli G, Becattini C, Meyer G, et al. Apixaban for the treatment of venous thromboembolism associated with cancer. N Engl J Med 2020;382(17): 1599–607.

120. Palareti G, Cosmi B, Lessiani G, et al. Evolution of untreated calf deep-vein thrombosis in high risk symptomatic outpatients: the blind, prospective CALTHRO study. Thromb Haemost 2010;104(5): 1063–70.

121. Righini M, Galanaud JP, Guenneguez H, et al. Anticoagulant therapy for symptomatic calf deep vein thrombosis (CACTUS): a randomised, double-blind, placebo-controlled trial. Lancet Haematol 2016;3(12):e556–62.

122. Robert-Ebadi H, Righini M. Management of distal deep vein thrombosis. Thromb Res 2017;149:48–55.

123. Galanaud JP, Genty C, Sevestre MA, et al. Predictive factors for concurrent deep-vein thrombosis and symptomatic venous thromboembolic recurrence in case of superficial venous thrombosis. The OPTIMEV study. Thromb Haemost 2011; 105(1):31–9.

124. Kahn SR, Ginsberg JS. The post-thrombotic syndrome: current knowledge, controversies, and directions for future research. Blood Rev 2002; 16(3):155–65.

125. O'Connell C. How I treat incidental pulmonary embolism. Blood 2015;125(12):1877–82 [quiz: 2009].

126. Baumann Kreuziger L, Jaffray J, Carrier M. Epidemiology, diagnosis, prevention and treatment of catheter-related thrombosis in children and adults. Thromb Res 2017;157:64–71.

127. Rajasekhar A, Streiff MB. How I treat central venous access device-related upper extremity deep vein thrombosis. Blood 2017;129(20):2727–36.

128. Martin K, Beyer-Westendorf J, Davidson BL, et al. Use of the direct oral anticoagulants in obese patients: guidance from the SSC of the ISTH. J Thromb Haemost 2016;14(6):1308–13.

129. Kido K, Lee JC, Hellwig T, et al. Use of direct oral anticoagulants in morbidly obese patients. Pharmacotherapy 2020;40(1):72–83.

130. Coons JC, Albert L, Bejjani A, et al. Effectiveness and safety of direct oral anticoagulants versus warfarin in obese patients with acute venous thromboembolism. Pharmacotherapy 2020;40(3):204–10.

131. Martin KA, Lee CR, Farrell TM, et al. Oral anticoagulant use after bariatric surgery: a literature review and clinical guidance. Am J Med 2017;130(5): 517–24.

132. Sista AK, Klok FA. Late outcomes of pulmonary embolism: the post-PE syndrome. Thromb Res 2018; 164:157–62.

133. Wilkens H, Konstantinides S, Lang IM, et al. Chronic thromboembolic pulmonary hypertension (CTEPH): updated recommendations from the Cologne Consensus Conference 2018. Int J Cardiol 2018;272s:69–78.

134. Pikovsky O, Rabinovich A. Prevention and treatment of the post-thrombotic syndrome. Thromb Res 2018;164:116–24.

135. Soosainathan A, Moore HM, Gohel MS, et al. Scoring systems for the post-thrombotic syndrome. J Vasc Surg 2013;57(1):254–61.

136. Kahn SR, Shapiro S, Wells PS, et al. Compression stockings to prevent post-thrombotic syndrome: a randomised placebo-controlled trial. Lancet 2014; 383(9920):880–8.

Varicose Veins and Chronic Venous Disease

Tom Alsaigh, MD, Eri Fukaya, MD, PhD*

KEYWORDS

- Chronic venous disease • Venous insufficiency • Varicose vein • Venous reflux

KEY POINTS

- Chronic venous disease is a growing worldwide problem associated with significant morbidity.
- Venous insufficiency results in increased ambulatory venous pressure and ultimately venous hypertension.
- The central principle in the conservative management of venous reflux is compression therapy.

INTRODUCTION

Chronic venous disease (CVD) is a growing worldwide problem associated with significant morbidity. It results from longstanding venous insufficiency and venous hypertension, and is manifested clinically by pain, edema, skin pigmentation, distended veins in the lower extremity, and ulceration of the skin in severe cases. Its pathophysiology involves a complex interplay of inflammation and tissue remodeling, and numerous technical advances have shaped current treatment. Here, we comprehensively review the anatomy, pathophysiology, genomics, clinical classification, and treatment modalities of CVD.

VENOUS ANATOMY

The venous system is a large conduit for blood return to the heart and is estimated to contain about 70% of the blood volume at any given time because of its high capacitance relative to its arterial counterpart.[1,2] It originates as capillaries, which become the venules and veins, as it increases in size. The lower extremity venous network consists of deep and superficial veins connected by perforators and contains intraluminal valves that help ensure unidirectional blood flow toward the heart. The largest axial superficial veins of the lower extremities include the great saphenous vein (GSV) and the small saphenous vein (SSV). The GSV courses in between the superficial and deep compartments separated by the saphenous fascia and resembles the so-called "Egyptian eye" on cross-sectional view in B-mode ultrasound.[3] It originates from where the dorsal vein of the hallux merges with the dorsal venous arch of the foot, passes in front of the medial malleolus of the foot, and courses up the medial side of the leg to join the common femoral vein at the saphenofemoral junction.[3] The SSV is located on the posterior aspect of the calf between the two heads of the gastrocnemius muscle and courses upward through the popliteal fossa, ultimately draining into the popliteal vein or continues cranially and empties into the femoral vein or the GSV more proximally.[4] The SSV lies in its own saphenous compartment, delineated by the superficial and muscular fascia.[4] Other axial veins coursing parallel to the GSV include anterior accessory GSV and the posterior accessory GSV.

Deep veins of the lower extremities begin by draining the foot at the deep plantar venous arch, which at the medial malleolus becomes the posterior tibial vein, whereas the dorsalis pedis vein on the dorsum of the foot becomes the anterior tibial vein at the ankle.[5] The tibioperoneal trunk and the anterior tibial veins join to form the popliteal vein, which courses cranially through the

The authors have nothing to disclose.
Division of Vascular Surgery, Vascular Medicine Section, Stanford University, 780 Welch Road, Suite CJ 350, Palo Alto, CA 94304, USA
* Corresponding author.
E-mail address: efukaya@stanford.edu

Cardiol Clin 39 (2021) 567–581
https://doi.org/10.1016/j.ccl.2021.06.009
0733-8651/21/© 2021 Elsevier Inc. All rights reserved.

adductor canal to become the femoral vein.[4] The femoral vein then joins with the deep femoral vein to become the common femoral vein.

Perforator veins penetrate the deep fascia to connect the deep and superficial veins and are often found in the medial calf and thigh. The perforator veins may connect the saphenous vein and the deep veins but can also arise and become superficial nonaxial tributary veins (**Fig. 1**).

EPIDEMIOLOGY

CVD is a common condition. The prevalence of CVD varies geographically, with reports of chronic venous insufficiency (CVI) found in up to 40% of women and 17% of men in Western countries.[6] Prevalence of varicose veins vary widely, which are reported in 1% to 73% of women and 2% to 56% of men.[6]

In the San Diego population study, ~30% of the population had varicose veins or lower extremity skin changes because of venous disease. More than 25% of the population had disease of either major superficial or deep veins in the leg.[7] The prevalence of varicose veins and CVI increases with age.[7] The Edinburgh Vein Study sought to determine the prevalence of varicose veins and CVI in men and women aged 18 to 64 years.[8] Although some studies have shown an increased prevalence of varicose veins and CVI in women compared with men,[9,10] this study found that prevalence of trunk varices was similar in both groups but CVI and mild varicose veins were more common in men than women.[8] This study highlights the geographic diversity, study methodology,

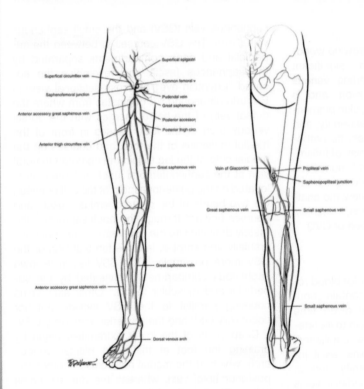

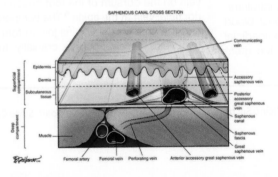

Fig. 1. Venous anatomy. (*From* Almeida J. Atlas of Endovascular Venous Surgery. Elsevier Saunders 2012 location 266, 285, 317; with permission. (Figure 1-3, 1-4, 1-5 in original).)

self-reporting of disease, and diagnostic imaging that may contribute to differences in disease epidemiology.

Increased age is associated with vessel wall and venous valve deterioration. In addition, weakening of the calf muscles can contribute to prolonged venous hypertension. Female gender is a risk factor, but it is unclear if this is driven by worsening CVD during pregnancy or other genetic, hormonal, or environmental factors. Obesity (body mass index >30 kg/m^2) is a significant predictor of clinically significant venous disease in both men and women,[11] and is associated with more significant skin changes and ulceration.[12] Family history is also a well-known contributing factor.[13,14] Data from the Swedish multigeneration registry showed that family history of hospital treatment for varicose veins was associated with an increased risk of similar treatment among relatives.[15] In a prospective, community-based study of half a million individuals using the UK Biobank and machine learning algorithms, Fukaya and colleagues[16] identified several known (age, sex, obesity, pregnancy, and history of deep vein thrombosis) and novel (leg bioimpedance and increased height) as risk factors for varicose vein development.

PATHOPHYSIOLOGY OF CLINICAL VENOUS DISEASE

The venous system is a large volume, low pressure, velocity, and resistance system that must overcome the hydrostatic pressure induced by gravity and the column of blood from the right atrium to the foot to effectively return the blood back to the heart. Venous valves are spread throughout the veins and help to prevent retrograde blood flow while also conducting blood from the superficial to the deep venous system.[17] In addition to vein valves, the calf muscle pump also provides pressure to assist venous return in the lower extremities against gravity. Thus, a higher degree of muscle activity, such as walking, can enhance venous emptying of the healthy human leg. A decrease in muscle activity and joint movement reduces the efficacy of the muscle-vein pump.[18] Contraction of the calf muscle increases the pressure in the deep venous compartment of the leg to about 140 mm Hg, thereby overcoming the hydrostatic pressure in the lower extremities and pushing blood from the superficial to the deep veins of the leg.[19] Physiologic reflux occurs during muscle relaxation, lasting about 0.2 to 0.3 seconds in veins with competent valves,[19,20] and sometimes slightly longer in the common femoral vein. Retrograde flow longer than 0.5 seconds in the superficial veins and 1.0 seconds in the deep veins on ultrasound examination defines venous incompetence.[4] Venous incompetence, venous insufficiency, and venous reflux are often used interchangeably to describe a phenomenon of valvular incompetence in the veins leading to venous hypertension. Venous insufficiency is characterized by decreased forward flow of blood from the lower extremities to the heart, thereby increasing ambulatory venous pressure and resulting in venous hypertension. Over time, the increased venous pressure results in further valve damage, inflammatory changes, and remodeling of the vessel wall, ultimately leading to CVD, with clinical manifestations including skin pigmentation and trophic changes, varicose veins, edema, and in severe cases skin ulceration.[21–25] Specifically, venous hypertension results in pressure elevation that leads to venous valve incompetence with resultant reflux, inflammation, and a microcirculatory pressure burden in the lower leg. The sustained inflammatory phase involves macrophages, neutrophils, and T-lymphocytes releasing cytokines that enhance the expression of adhesion molecules such as ICAM-1, VCAM, LFA-1, and VLA-4, ultimately leading to more leukocyte infiltration and inflammation.[26–28] Increased proteolytic activity by MMPs and decreased activity by tissue inhibitors of MMPs (TIMPs) also help to remodel the ulcer microenvironment and contribute to disease pathogenesis[28] (**Fig. 2**).

The etiology of CVD is related to either primary valvular insufficiency or secondary to post-thrombotic syndrome (PTS), which is caused by intravenous obstruction after deep venous thrombosis (DVT), extrinsic venous compression, or pelvic congestion syndrome. Most cases of valvular insufficiency are multifactorial with underlying predisposition in patients who have a family history of venous disease, obesity, advanced age, prolonged standing, female gender, pregnancy, and hormonal changes. In some cases, valve incompetence may be congenital (ie, Klippel-Trenaunay Syndrome), or result from trauma or thrombosis.[29] Venous obstruction due to DVT is an important cause of CVD and may lead to PTS with symptoms of leg heaviness, pain, cramping, swelling, and/or discoloration. PTS can develop in 20% to 50% of patients within 1 to 2 years of symptomatic DVT. A severe form of PTS manifests as ulceration (**Fig. 3**), in one-quarter to one-third of patients with PTS.[30,31] DVT in the iliac, femoral, popliteal, and calf veins can all lead to PTS.

Iliocaval venous obstruction (ICVO) represents central venous obstruction, which may contribute to venous hypertension and insufficiency. Etiologies of ICVO may be classified as nonthrombotic

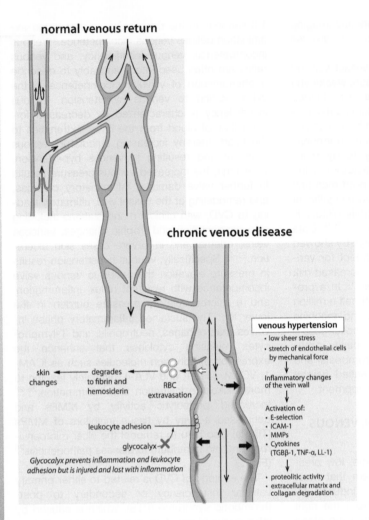

normal venous return

chronic venous disease

venous hypertension
- low sheer stress
- stretch of endothelial cells by mechanical force

Inflammatory changes of the vein wall

Activation of:
- E-selection
- ICAM-1
- MMPs
- Cytokines (TGBβ-1, TNF-α, LL-1)

- proteolitic activity
- extracellular matrix and collagan degradation

skin changes ← degrades to fibrin and hemosiderin ← RBC extravasation

leukocyte adhesion

glycocalyx

Glycocalyx prevents inflammation and leukocyte adhesion but is injured and lost with inflammation

Fig. 2. Chronic venous disease pathology. (*From* Baylis RA, Smith NL, Klarin D, Fukaya E. Epidemiology and Genetics of Venous Thromboembolism and Chronic Venous Disease. Circ Res. 2021 Jun 11;128(12):1988-2002; with permission. (Figure 1 in original).)

or thrombotic. The most common nonthrombotic cause is May-Thurner syndrome, which refers to obstruction of the left iliac vein by the overlying right common iliac artery.[32] Importantly, extrinsic compression by tumors,[33] renal,[34] or hepatic[35] cysts may also cause ICVO. Thrombotic occlusion occurs due to DVT, which may be due to inherited thrombophilia, acquired hypercoagulability, or IVC filter placement.[36] The initial imaging study for evaluation of ICVO is duplex venous ultrasound, followed by CT or MR venography and intravascular ultrasound (IVUS) if intervention is planned. Depending on etiology and symptoms, treatment may be conservative (compression and anticoagulation), or require endovascular intervention with angioplasty and stenting or open surgical and hybrid reconstructions.[37,38]

Pelvic congestion syndrome occurs in up to 4% of women and is characterized by chronic pelvic/vulvar discomfort, dyspareunia, abdominal bloating, pressure, and swelling worsened by prolonged standing, exercise, and coitus in women who have ovarian vein reflux and periovarian varicosities.[39] Because the perineal veins of female external genitalia do not have valves, they are susceptible to the development of varices, especially during pregnancy. Vulvar varicosities may occur due to GSV incompetence or insufficiency of the internal iliac and ovarian veins.[40] If symptoms of discomfort are severe, treatment may include ovarian vein embolization and coiling or sclerotherapy,[41] with the decision algorithm for who and when to treat being beyond the scope of this article.

GENOMICS

The importance of genetics and heritability of varicose veins and CVI has long been postulated based on familial studies.[42] Genes and proteins identified in CVD pathogenesis through candidate gene studies include connexins, such as Cx37, which are critical for proper venous valve

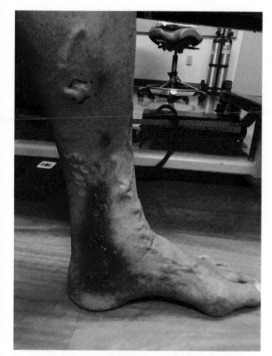

Fig. 3. Skin changes and ulcer due to post-thrombotic syndrome.

development[43]; matrix gla protein (MGP), which is an extracellular matrix remodeling protein that is, increased in varicose veins[44]; and the FOXC2 gene, which encodes a regulatory transcription factor involved in lymphatic and vascular development[45] and is associated with venous valve failure and reflux.[46]

More recent efforts have used genome-wide association studies (GWAS) to identify common genetic variants that confer susceptibility to CVD.[47] Ellinghaus and colleagues identified 3 novel CVD susceptibility loci, including *EFEMP1* (fibulin-3, an extracellular matrix glycoprotein), *KCNH8* (member of the human Elk voltage-gated potassium channel), and *SKAP2* (adaptor protein involved in Src signaling). Varicose veins, a common manifestation of prolonged venous reflux, have been subjected to genomics analyses as well. Fukaya and colleagues evaluated GWAS data from the UK Biobank to identify genetic variants that influence varicose vein susceptibility and identified 855 new SNPs associated with varicose veins that exceeded genome-wide significance. Critical variants identified include *CASZ1* gene on chromosome 1 (known blood pressure locus), *PIEZO1*, and *GALNS*. In addition, eQTL analyses identified several genes significantly regulated by the varicose vein SNPs to affect vascular development and skeletal abnormalities. These loci are involved in pathways of vascular development and skeletal/limb biology.

CLINICAL EXAMINATION

The history and physical examination are critical for the evaluation of CVD. Patients with CVD typically complain of leg swelling, pain, heaviness aggravated by prolonged standing and alleviated by leg elevation, skin itching, burning or irritation, throbbing and aching, and cramping.[48] Symptoms typically worsen toward the end of the day and are relieved with compression, elevation, and exercise. Patients should be asked about family history, occupation, exercise habits, changes in weight, use of compression socks and garments, thromboembolic history, allergies, medications that can predispose to DVT or lower extremity swelling, pregnancy history, and cardiac, renal, and other comorbidities.[49]

The physical examination for a CVD patient should be performed while the patient is standing, with both legs fully exposed. The lower extremities should be examined for distribution of varicosities, edema, skin changes, and limb size discrepancies. Especially for elderly patients who have bilateral edema, it is important to examine their gait, calf muscle function, and ankle and foot mobility. Individuals should be asked about prolonged sitting time with legs in a dependent position, and whether they sleep in a bed versus a recliner. Skin changes associated with CVD include hemosiderin deposits causing hyperpigmentation, and lipodermatosclerosis, which causes hardening of the skin, often with a bark-like shiny appearance resulting in an inverted champagne bottle-like appearance with a band-like stricture around the ankle (**Fig. 4**). Prolonged venous hypertension can predispose to recurrent cellulitis causing erythema and induration around the gaitor area. It is not unusual to see dilated veins around the ankles, otherwise known as corona phlebectatica (**Fig. 5**), not to be confused with regular spider or reticular veins. Venous leg ulcers (either active or healed) can frequently be seen in advanced venous disease.

The abdomen, flank, and pubis should be examined for the presence of venous collaterals, which is pathognomonic of iliac or iliocaval outflow obstruction.[4]

The differential diagnosis of CVD includes arterial, neurologic, rheumatologic, orthopedic disease, or congenital vascular malformation. In all cases, an effort should be made to measure thigh, calf, or another limb circumference for follow-up comparison.

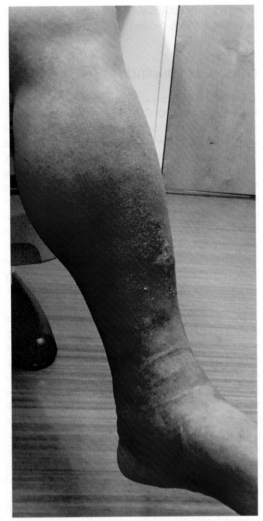

Fig. 4. Lipodermatosclerosis with inverted champagne bottle-like appearance.

CLINICAL-ETIOLOGICAL-ANATOMICAL-PATHOPHYSIOLOGICAL CLASSIFICATION

Standardized reporting of CVD manifestation occurs via the clinical-etiological-anatomical-pathophysiological (CEAP) classification, which was first assembled by the American Venous Forum in 1994.

The clinical (C) classification is scored from 0 (no evidence of venous disease) to 6 (active ulceration).[50] Major updates were added to the classification system in 2020,[50] which made it more detailed in depicting the venous pathophysiology, but also more difficult to use because of its complexity (**Table 1**). Among the revisions to the clinical (C) classification include the addition of a subscript 'r' for recurrent disease in C2 (varicose veins) and C6 (venous ulcers) classes. The

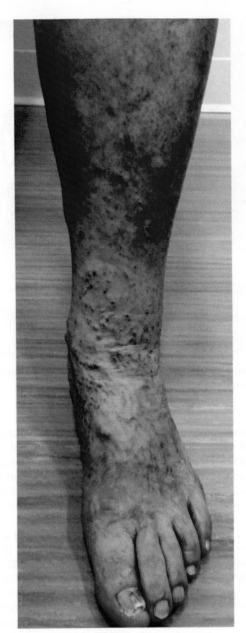

Fig. 5. Corona phlebectatica.

rationale for this addition is that some cases of disease recurrence may require different treatment strategies. The other revision in the clinical classification includes the addition of corona phlebectatica to the C4 class, in addition to its subdivision into 3 categories: C4a, C4b, and C4c. Corona phlebectatica is defined as a fan-shaped pattern of numerous small intradermal veins on the medial or lateral aspects of the foot and ankle, and may be an early sign of advanced venous disease,[50] as these patients were shown to be 5 times more likely to develop an ulcer.[51]

Table 1
Clinical classification of CEAP

Updated CEAP Classification System (2020)	
C0	No visible or palpable signs of venous disease
C1	Telangiectasias or reticular veins
C2	Varicose veins
C2r	Recurrent varicose veins
C3	Edema
C4	Changes in skin and subcutaneous tissue secondary to CVD
C4a	Pigmentation or eczema
C4b	Lipodermatosclerosis or atrophie blanche
C4c	Corona phlebectatica
C5	Healed venous ulcer
C6	Active venous ulcer
C6r	Recurrent active venous ulcer

One consequence of prolonged venous reflux is the development of lower extremity ulcers. Venous ulcers tend to occur around the medial malleolus and are associated with pain that improves with elevation, edema, and localized skin pigmentation. Open venous ulcers occur in about 0.3% of the adult population while a history of open or healed ulceration occurs in around 1%.[52] Approximately, 20% of people with CVI develop venous ulcers.[53]

Risk factors for ulcer recurrence include prolonged ulcer healing time (greater than 3 months), superficial venous reflux, PTS, deep vein occlusion, incompetent perforators, venous axial reflux, and higher ambulatory venous pressure.[54–56] Appropriate evaluation, monitoring, and treatment of venous ulcers is crucial to heal ulcers and prevent their recurrence.

Although ulcer healing is achievable with correct therapy, ulcer recurrence is a significant problem,[54] as up to 40% of patients with venous leg ulcers have frequent recurrences.[57] In the United States, more than 20,000 new patients are diagnosed with a venous ulcer each year,[58] direct medical costs are estimated at up to $1 billion annually, and the annual US payor burden is estimated at $14.9 billion.[58–60]

The etiology (E) classification represents the etiology of venous disease and is separated into congenital (Ec), primary (Ep), and secondary or post-thrombotic (Es) categories.[50] Although the definitions of the E subclasses have been refined, there have been no major changes to the previous version.[50]

The anatomic (A) classification of venous disease is described as superficial (A$_S$), deep (A$_D$), or perforating (A$_P$) veins. Replacing numeric descriptions of the venous segments by their common abbreviations, the 2020 classification scheme allows for a more intuitive identification of these anatomic segments.

The pathophysiologic (P) classification has basic designations including reflux (r), obstruction (o), reflux and obstruction (r,o), and no venous pathophysiology (n), as well as advanced designations, which are the same as previous with the addition of any of the named specific A anatomic venous segments.[50]

Because of its descriptive nature and use as a purely static categorical classification scheme, CEAP is also accompanied by the venous clinical severity score (VCSS), which was developed as an evaluation tool that would be responsive to changes in disease severity over time and in response to treatment.[61] The widely used revised VCSS includes 9 hallmarks of venous disease scored on a severity scale from 0 to 3, with scores from 0 to 1 representing mild, 2 moderate, and 3 severe symptoms. The scored hallmarks include pain, edema, skin changes and pigmentation, inflammation and induration, as well as ulcers (number, size, and duration) and other parameters.[61]

NONINVASIVE IMAGING AND DIAGNOSTICS

Evaluation of venous disease at its earliest stages ensures timely treatment. Noninvasive methods to assess lower extremity hemodynamics is central to the diagnosis and management of venous disease. Duplex ultrasound is a sensitive diagnostic method[62] that combines B-mode imaging, continuous wave (CW), and pulsed wave (PW) Doppler modes to provide assessment of anatomy and hemodynamic function.[63] Blood vessel 2D structure may be imaged in the grayscale B-mode (brightness mode),[64] and blood flow evaluated in the Doppler mode. Noncompressibility of veins on grayscale imaging is highly sensitive and specific for the detection of DVT when compared with venography.[65] Grayscale imaging may also visualize venous valves, wall thickening, residual thrombus, and synechiae. The combination of CW and PW Doppler are used to assess venous blood flow. Flow patterns in relation to respiration are important to evaluate for venous disease since the loss of respiratory phasicity or pulsatile flow patterns can help identify the underlying pathology. Maneuvers to elicit venous reflux such as manual limb compression proximal or distal to the ultrasound probe or Valsalva provide information about retrograde blood flow and reflux[66] (Fig. 6).

Ultrasound should be performed with the patient either in the standing position or in steep reverse Trendelenburg to mimic the effect of gravity and the physiology seen in venous insufficiency.[67]

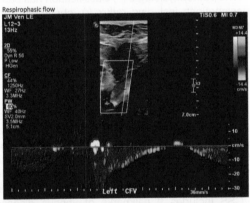

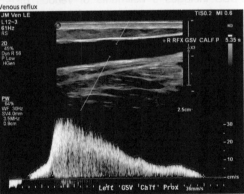

Fig. 6. Ultrasound images for respirophasic waveforms and venous reflux waveforms.

Visualization can be achieved as proximal as the external iliac veins, and the deep and superficial veins are evaluated for flow patterns, thrombus, and reflux. The evaluation for CVI starts just proximal to the saphenofemoral junction at the common femoral vein. The entire lower extremity should be imaged, including the greater saphenous vein (GSV), SSV, perforators, and deep veins. Normal superficial and deep veins should be completely compressible, display spontaneous flow at quiescence with no flow disturbance, and phasicity with respiratory variation (ie, decreased flow velocity with inspiration and an increase with expiration). A prompt increase in venous flow velocity is noted at a given location with distal augmentation, and valvular competence is indicated by cephalad, unidirectional flow with no retrograde flow.[52] A reversal of flow during diagnostic maneuvers suggests venous reflux, with physiologically significant reflux measuring around 0.5 seconds in the superficial veins or greater than 1 second in the femoral and popliteal veins.[53,66]

Imaging of the abdominal and pelvic veins should be performed with venography, as windows are limited with duplex ultrasound. Magnetic resonance venography and computed tomography venography offer sophisticated 3D reconstructions of the venous system, which help to identify iliocaval and pelvic venous pathologies such as May-Thurner syndrome, Nutcracker syndrome, or post-thrombotic obstruction.[68,69] Conventional venography and IVUS may be used in conjunction with these techniques for evaluation of iliac venous compression and outflow obstruction, and is used for assistance with placement of venous stents after venoplasty.[70]

TREATMENT MODALITIES

CVD treatment has long historical recognition. Hippocrates described the relationship between varicose veins and ulceration, as well as using compression therapy with layered bandages for treatment.[71] Physicians such as Celcus and Galen performed operations for varicose veins in the Roman era using blunt hooks for avulsion, which would be equivalent to the modern-day phlebectomy. In the late 19th century, Friedrich Trendelenburg reported on GSV ligation in the mid-thigh, which was the start of venous surgery.[72] The first stripping procedures were performed in the early 20th century and high ligation and/or stripping was the most common form of vein surgery until endovenous treatments became available in the past 20 years. Sclerotherapy has been used in venous therapies with different sclerosants since the 1950s.[73]

The goal in the treatment of CVD can include the following: (1) treatment of symptoms, (2) treatment of advanced CVD (treatment and prevention of recurrent venous ulceration), or (3) esthetic treatment of asymptomatic (C1 and C2) disease. The management of symptomatic and advanced CVD is considered medical treatment, whereas that for C1 and C2 is mostly considered cosmetic treatment, with some variable overlap. Treatment modalities for CVD include conservative therapies (compression), venotonic medications, and venous procedures including sclerotherapy, surgical therapy, and endovenous therapies.

Compression Therapy

The central principle in the conservative management of venous reflux is compression therapy, which serves to counteract the hydrostatic pressure exerted on the venous circulation from incompetent valves and other causes of venous hypertension, thereby reducing edema.[74] Compression is used to treat a wide range of CVD pathology, including swelling, symptomatic varicose veins, and venous ulcers. The Society of Vascular Surgery and American Venous Forum guidelines classify compression therapy as a grade IA recommendation for the treatment of CVD and VLUs.[57] Compression therapy improves healing in patients with venous ulceration.[75] In CVI-related lymphedema (or phlebolymphedema[76]), advanced pneumatic compression devices have proven effective at reducing annual hospitalizations, as well as total inpatient and outpatient costs.[76] Most common forms of compression used for therapy include elastic leg stockings, elastic and nonelastic multilayer wraps, and intermittent pneumatic compression (IPC).[4] IPC is a mechanical method of delivering compression to swollen limbs by applying a multi-chamber compression sleeve over the affected limb and sequentially inflating and deflating the device to apply sustained pressure, proving a venous milking effect. A meta-analysis of studies testing whether IPC improves leg venous ulcer healing suggests in one trial that ulcers healed more with IPC (62%) than with dressings alone (28%), and it remains inconclusive whether IPC increases healing when added to treatment with bandages or when used instead of compression bandages.[77] For patients with venous wounds, zinc oxide dressings are superior to alginates and are considered first-line to promote venous wound healing.[78] The Unna boot dressing is a compression method using a zinc oxide dressing in addition to nonelastic bandages that provide sufficient pressure both with activity and at rest and accelerates the venous ulcer healing process.[79]

Medical Therapy

Although there is no standard medical therapy for venous disease, there are a variety of venotonics used around the world for symptomatic alleviation. Diosmiplex is a micronized purified flavonoid fraction and has been used to prevent endothelial activation and inflammation, thereby slowing venous reflux and its clinical sequelae such as leg heaviness, swelling, and cramps.[80,81] Clinical trials have suggested that horse chestnut seed extract is an effective means of reducing edema, pain, and itching.[82]

Sclerotherapy

Sclerotherapy is an effective method to destroy and close incompetent veins. It involves injection of a chemical agent into the lumen of a vessel to induce damage and occlusion of the vessel. Vein sclerosing is achieved through direct injection of a liquid or foamed agent to provoke endothelial cell and vessel wall damage.[83] The goal is to deliver a minimum volume and concentration that will cause irreversible damage while leaving adjacent normal vessels untouched. There are several types of sclerosing solutions. The detergent solutions, sodium tetradecyl sulfate and polidocanol, attack endothelial cells at their cell surface lipids. The hyperosmolar/hypertonic solution (hypertonic saline, hypertonic dextrose, and sodium salicylate) destroys endothelial cells via dehydration. Glycerin acts as a chemical irritant through its caustic effects on the endothelium.

Foam sclerotherapy is a form of treatment for varicose veins, incompetent veins, reticular veins, and spider veins, and has become increasingly popular, as foam displaces intravascular blood and is not diluted in it, keeping the intravascular concentration of the sclerosing agent known and controlled.[83,84] Through foaming, a smaller quantity of sclerosing agent leads to the homogenous distribution of sclerosant in the vessel lumen, thereby increasing the surface area contact of the therapeutic with the endothelium. Foam is also quite stable and only a short amount of contact time with the vessel is required to provide an adequate therapeutic effect.[85] Because the foam is created by mixing gas bubbles with the sclerosing agent, the resultant product has echogenicity and can act as an excellent contrast medium when being injected under ultrasound guidance.

The DSS or Tessari method is often used for physician compounded foam. This can be done with room air, although some voice concern that the use of room air to compound foam increases the risk of embolization to the brain because of the high nitrogen content. The ideal bubble size should be under 100 μm to prevent adverse events related to the use of foam-related air embolism, which with a patent foramen ovale (PFO) can cause stroke, seizure, transient ischemic attacks, or myocardial infarction.[86]

Polidocanol is among the most widely used sclerosants and is very well-tolerated. Contraindications for its use include allergy, presence of acute or superficial DVT, advanced PAD, first trimester and late (>36 weeks) pregnancy, and immobility.[83,87] Complications from polidocanol foam sclerotherapy include urtication, hyperpigmentation, telangiectatic matting along the inner thigh, calves, and ankles, and rarer side effects include those associated with PFO.[83,88,89]

Endovenous Treatment

Catheter-based treatments used to cause occlusion of incompetent veins include thermal and nonthermal ablation options. Endovenous thermal ablation uses ultrasound-guided, catheter-directed thermal energy within incompetent veins to cause endothelial damage, causing the vein wall to contract and occlude, thereby shunting blood to other tributary veins and pathways. The two prominent methods are endovenous laser ablation (EVLA) and radiofrequency ablation (RFA). In both techniques, ablation starts about 2 to 3 cm distal to the saphenofemoral junction, and a tumescent liquid is injected around the saphenous vein for anesthesia and to prevent heat dispersion. EVLA involves the transmission of laser energy within an optical fiber placed within the vein. This energy is then absorbed by hemoglobin or water within the vessel, creating heat and ultimately vessel damage leading to occlusion.[90] RFA involves the use of a catheter-mounted electrode that is, introduced into the vein, after which an electrical current is passed through a metal coil at the tip of the catheter, thereby applying heat directly to the vein wall.[90] Endovenous thermal ablations are the treatment of choice for saphenous incompetence, and most current evidence supports ablation of an incompetent superficial venous system to promote ulcer healing and prevent ulcer.[91,92] The EVRA-Ulcer trial was a multicenter randomized controlled trial (RCT), which sought to delineate whether compression therapy alone or combined with endovenous ablation of superficial venous reflux was more efficacious for venous leg ulcer healing.[93] The results showed that the time to ulcer healing was shorter in the early intervention

compared with the deferred treatment group, with a median time to ulcer healing of 56 days (95% confidence interval [CI], 49–66) in the early intervention group and 82 days (95% CI, 69–92) in the deferred intervention group.[93] In addition, early endovenous ablation provided a longer time free from ulceration. Endothermal heat-induced thrombosis occurs in up to 3% of cases of thermal ablation,[94] and depending on severity, may be treated with observation, antiplatelet therapy, or full-dose anticoagulation.[95]

Treatment of GSV reflux with EVLA, RFA, ultrasound-guided foam sclerotherapy, or surgical vein stripping was evaluated one RCT.[96] Although all treatments were efficacious, the technical failure rate was highest with foam sclerotherapy. Notably, RFA and foam were associated with a faster recovery and less postoperative pain than EVLA and stripping.

The nonthermal, nontumescent endovenous treatment includes the use of cyanoacrylate glue and mechanochemical ablation. The VenaSeal (Medtronic, MN) technology dispenses cyanoacrylate glue from the catheter tip to occlude or "seal" the refluxing truncal superficial veins.[97] This has a comparable closure rate to RFA and can avoid some adverse effects associated with thermal techniques such as endothermal heat-induced thrombosis and discomfort due to infiltration of tumescent fluid.[98] However, the implant of a glue polymer may occasionally cause hypersensitivity or an allergic reaction[99] or foreign body granulomas.[100,101]

Mechanochemical endovenous ablation uses a rotating wire within a catheter to mechanically damage the endothelium of a vessel, while at the same time, a sclerosant is infused at the end of the catheter, which causes chemical damage to the same segment of the vein wall.[102] Mechanochemical ablation of the GSV was shown to be safe and effective,[103] with no major complications such as DVT, pulmonary embolism, or nerve injury reported in several trials.[104,105]

Percutaneous transluminal angioplasty is an endovenous treatment of ICVO, which involves traversing the obstruction with a guidewire, followed by the deployment of a venous stent to cover the obstructed vein segment.[106] With the recent emergence of new venous stents, multiple clinical trials are ongoing to evaluate the use of this in ICVO[107–109] and although it is likely that this may benefit a subpopulation of these patients, it is important to realize that the current quality of evidence supporting venous stenting of the lower extremity is from clinical trials that are not randomized and there is still lack of guidelines or indications for the appropriate use of these stents.

Surgical Treatment

For surgical treatment of uncomplicated varicose veins, high ligation or high ligation with stripping of the saphenous vein have been used. High ligation refers to surgically tying off a vein to prevent blood flow into a diseased vein. With recent advances in endovenous therapy, these techniques are used mostly in cases when there is a contraindication to endovenous treatment. For example, stripping may be performed when there is a significant thrombus in the vein that precludes the passing of a catheter through the lumen. RCTs comparing mostly with EVLA, RFA, and foam sclerotherapy showed that all therapies are effective in improving VCSS and quality of life. However, increased rates of recanalization and reoperation are seen after foam sclerotherapy.[110]

Ambulatory phlebectomy is a safe and effective procedure that includes removal or avulsion of varicose veins through small incisions in the leg, and can be performed under local anesthesia in an office setting.[111] It should be considered as an adjunct treatment to endovenous ablation of the main refluxing truncal vein,[112] or a procedure to independently remove varicose veins.[113]

SUMMARY

The growing prevalence of venous disease in an aging population will consequently lead to a greater economic burden on individuals and health care systems. In addition to economic consequences, quality of life suffers in patients with CVD. It is critical for clinicians to recognize venous disease early in its course and facilitate close monitoring and follow-up to ensure timely treatment. Continued emphasis on basic mechanisms of disease progression is important and may help facilitate the development of novel pharmacotherapies for venous disease, which may be used in lieu of, or in combination with interventional therapies discussed in this review.

CLINICS CARE POINTS

- Venous hypertension results in chronic venous disease with clinical manifestations including skin pigmentation, varicose veins, edema, and in severe cases skin ulceration.
- Deep venous thrombosis can cause of chronic venous disease and post thrombotic syndrome.

- Pelvic congestion syndrome can occur in women who have ovarian vein reflux and periovarian varicosities.
- Duplex ultrasound examination is central to diagnosis and management of venous disease.
- Treatment modalities for CVD includes compression therapy medications, and venous procedures.

REFERENCES

1. Meissner MH, Moneta G, Burnand K, et al. The hemodynamics and diagnosis of venous disease. J Vasc Surg 2007;46(Suppl S):4s–24s.
2. Swift MR, Weinstein BM. Arterial-venous specification during development. Circ Res 2009;104(5):576–88.
3. Caggiati A. The saphenous venous compartments. Surg Radiol Anat 1999;21(1):29–34.
4. Wittens C, Davies AH, Bækgaard N, et al. Editor's choice - management of chronic venous disease: clinical practice guidelines of the European Society for Vascular Surgery (ESVS). Eur J Vasc Endovasc Surg 2015;49(6):678–737.
5. White JV, Katz ML, Cisek P, et al. Venous outflow of the leg: anatomy and physiologic mechanism of the plantar venous plexus. J Vasc Surg 1996;24(5):819–24.
6. Beebe-Dimmer JL, Pfeifer JR, Engle JS, et al. The epidemiology of chronic venous insufficiency and varicose veins. Ann Epidemiol 2005;15(3):175–84.
7. Criqui MH, Jamosmos M, Fronek A, et al. Chronic venous disease in an ethnically diverse population: the San Diego Population Study. Am J Epidemiol 2003;158(5):448–56.
8. Evans CJ, Fowkes FG, Ruckley CV, et al. Prevalence of varicose veins and chronic venous insufficiency in men and women in the general population: Edinburgh Vein Study. J Epidemiol Community Health 1999;53(3):149–53.
9. Vuylsteke ME, Colman R, Thomis S, et al. The influence of age and gender on venous symptomatology. An epidemiological survey in Belgium and Luxembourg. Phlebology 2016;31(5):325–33.
10. Vuylsteke ME, Thomis S, Guillaume G, et al. Epidemiological study on chronic venous disease in Belgium and Luxembourg: prevalence, risk factors, and symptomatology. Eur J Vasc Endovasc Surg 2015;49(4):432–9.
11. Padberg F Jr, Cerveira JJ, Lal BK, et al. Does severe venous insufficiency have a different etiology in the morbidly obese? Is it venous? J Vasc Surg 2003;37(1):79–85.

12. Danielsson G, Eklof B, Grandinetti A, et al. The influence of obesity on chronic venous disease. Vasc Endovascular Surg 2002;36(4):271–6.

13. Serra R, Buffone G, de Franciscis A, et al. A genetic study of chronic venous insufficiency. Ann Vasc Surg 2012;26(5):636–42.

14. Anwar MA, Georgiadis KA, Shalhoub J, et al. A review of familial, genetic, and congenital aspects of primary varicose vein disease. Circ Cardiovasc Genet 2012;5(4):460–6.

15. Zöller B, Ji J, Sundquist J, et al. Family history and risk of hospital treatment for varicose veins in Sweden. Br J Surg 2012;99(7):948–53.

16. Fukaya E, Flores AM, Lindholm D, et al. Clinical and genetic determinants of varicose veins. Circulation 2018;138(25):2869–80.

17. Goldman MP, Fronek A. Anatomy and pathophysiology of varicose veins. J Dermatol Surg Oncol 1989;15(2):138–45.

18. Kugler C, Strunk M, Rudofsky G. Venous pressure dynamics of the healthy human leg. Role of muscle activity, joint mobility and anthropometric factors. J Vasc Res 2001;38(1):20–9.

19. Baliyan V, Tajmir S, Hedgire SS, et al. Lower extremity venous reflux. Cardiovasc Diagn Ther 2016;6(6):533–43.

20. Arnoldi CC. Venous pressure in the leg of healthy human subjects at rest and during muscular exercise in the nearly erect position. Acta Chir Scand 1965;130(6):570–83.

21. Xie T, Ye J, Rerkasem K, et al. The venous ulcer continues to be a clinical challenge: an update. Burns Trauma 2018;6:18.

22. Falanga V, Eaglstein WH. The "trap" hypothesis of venous ulceration. Lancet 1993;341(8851):1006–8.

23. Schmid-Schönbein GW, Takase S, Bergan JJ. New advances in the understanding of the pathophysiology of chronic venous insufficiency. Angiology 2001;52(Suppl 1):S27–34.

24. Bergan JJ, Schmid-Schönbein GW, Smith PD, et al. Chronic venous disease. N Engl J Med 2006;355(5):488–98.

25. Anwar MA, Shalhoub J, Lim CS, et al. The effect of pressure-induced mechanical stretch on vascular wall differential gene expression. J Vasc Res 2012;49(6):463–78.

26. Simka M. Cellular and molecular mechanisms of venous leg ulcers development–the "puzzle" theory. Int Angiol 2010;29(1):1–19.

27. Moore K, Huddleston E, Stacey MC, et al. Venous leg ulcers - the search for a prognostic indicator. Int Wound J 2007;4(2):163–72.

28. Raffetto JD, Ligi D, Maniscalco R, et al. Why venous leg ulcers have difficulty healing: overview on pathophysiology, clinical consequences, and treatment. J Clin Med 2020;10(1):29.

29. Mutlak O, Aslam M, Standfield NJ. Chronic venous insufficiency: a new concept to understand pathophysiology at the microvascular level - a pilot study. Perfusion 2019;34(1):84–9.

30. Prandoni P, Lensing AW, Cogo A, et al. The long-term clinical course of acute deep venous thrombosis. Ann Intern Med 1996;125(1):1–7.

31. Brandjes DP, Buller HR, Heijboer H, et al. Randomised trial of effect of compression stockings in patients with symptomatic proximal-vein thrombosis. Lancet 1997;349(9054):759–62.

32. Liddell RP, Evans NS. May-Thurner syndrome. Vasc Med 2018;23(5):493–6.

33. Goel S, Gupta AK, Goel A, et al. IVC tumoural thrombosis: an unusual complication of testicular tumour. BMJ Case Rep 2017;2017. bcr2017220677.

34. O'Sullivan DA, Torres VE, Heit JA, et al. Compression of the inferior vena cava by right renal cysts: an unusual cause of IVC and/or iliofemoral thrombosis with pulmonary embolism in autosomal dominant polycystic kidney disease. Clin Nephrol 1998;49(5):332–4.

35. Iguchi S, Kasai A, Kishimoto H, et al. Thrombosis in inferior vena cava (IVC) due to intra-cystic hemorrhage into a hepatic local cyst with autosomal dominant polycystic kidney disease (ADPKD). Intern Med 2004;43(3):209–12.

36. Gorman PH, Qadri SF, Rao-Patel A. Prophylactic inferior vena cava (IVC) filter placement may increase the relative risk of deep venous thrombosis after acute spinal cord injury. J Trauma 2009;66(3):707–12.

37. Schleimer K, Barbati ME, Grommes J, et al. Update on diagnosis and treatment strategies in patients with post-thrombotic syndrome due to chronic venous obstruction and role of endovenous recanalization. J Vasc Surg Venous Lymphat Disord 2019;7(4):592–600.

38. Garg N, Gloviczki P, Karimi KM, et al. Factors affecting outcome of open and hybrid reconstructions for nonmalignant obstruction of iliofemoral veins and inferior vena cava. J Vasc Surg 2011;53(2):383–93.

39. Hobbs JT. The pelvic congestion syndrome. Br J Hosp Med 1990;43(3):200–6.

40. Scultetus AH, Villavicencio JL, Gillespie DL, et al. The pelvic venous syndromes: analysis of our experience with 57 patients. J Vasc Surg 2002;36(5):881–8.

41. O'Brien MT, Gillespie DL. Diagnosis and treatment of the pelvic congestion syndrome. J Vasc Surg Venous Lymphat Disord 2015;3(1):96–106.

42. Brinsuk M, Tank J, Luft FC, et al. Heritability of venous function in humans. Arterioscler Thromb Vasc Biol 2004;24(1):207–11.

43. Munger SJ, Kanady JD, Simon AM. Absence of venous valves in mice lacking Connexin37. Dev Biol 2013;373(2):338–48.

44. Cario-Toumaniantz C, Boularan C, Schurgers LJ, et al. Identification of differentially expressed genes in human varicose veins: involvement of matrix gla protein in extracellular matrix remodeling. J Vasc Res 2007;44(6):444–59.

45. Mellor RH, Brice G, Stanton AW, et al. Mutations in FOXC2 are strongly associated with primary valve failure in veins of the lower limb. Circulation 2007; 115(14):1912–20.

46. Pocock ES, Alsaigh T, Mazor R, et al. Cellular and molecular basis of venous insufficiency. Vasc Cell 2014;6(1):24.

47. Ellinghaus E, Ellinghaus D, Krusche P, et al. Genome-wide association analysis for chronic venous disease identifies EFEMP1 and KCNH8 as susceptibility loci. Sci Rep 2017;7(1):45652.

48. Santler B, Goerge T. Chronic venous insufficiency - a review of pathophysiology, diagnosis, and treatment. J Dtsch Dermatol Ges 2017;15(5):538–56.

49. Gloviczki P, Comerota AJ, Dalsing MC, et al. The care of patients with varicose veins and associated chronic venous diseases: clinical practice guidelines of the Society for Vascular Surgery and the American Venous Forum. J Vasc Surg 2011;53(5 Suppl):2s–48s.

50. Lurie F, Passman M, Meisner M, et al. The 2020 update of the CEAP classification system and reporting standards. J Vasc Surg Venous Lymphat Disord 2020;8(3):342–52.

51. Robertson L, Lee AJ, Gallagher K, et al. Risk factors for chronic ulceration in patients with varicose veins: a case control study. J Vasc Surg 2009; 49(6):1490–8.

52. Necas M. Duplex ultrasound in the assessment of lower extremity venous insufficiency. Australas J Ultrasound Med 2010;13(4):37–45.

53. Malgor RD, Labropoulos N. Diagnosis of venous disease with duplex ultrasound. Phlebology 2013; 28(Suppl 1):158–61.

54. Gloviczki P, Gloviczki ML. Evidence on efficacy of treatments of venous ulcers and on prevention of ulcer recurrence. Perspect Vasc Surg Endovasc Ther 2009;21(4):259–68.

55. Magnusson MB, Nelzén O, Volkmann R. Leg ulcer recurrence and its risk factors: a duplex ultrasound study before and after vein surgery. Eur J Vasc Endovasc Surg 2006;32(4):453–61.

56. Tenbrook JA Jr, Iafrati MD, O'Donnell TF Jr, et al. Systematic review of outcomes after surgical management of venous disease incorporating subfascial endoscopic perforator surgery. J Vasc Surg 2004;39(3):583–9.

57. O'Donnell TF Jr, Passman MA, Marston WA, et al. Management of venous leg ulcers: clinical practice guidelines of the Society for Vascular Surgery (R) and the American Venous Forum. J Vasc Surg 2014;60(2 Suppl):3S–59S.

58. Heit JA, Rooke TW, Silverstein MD, et al. Trends in the incidence of venous stasis syndrome and venous ulcer: a 25-year population-based study. J Vasc Surg 2001;33(5):1022–7.

59. Olin JW, Beusterien KM, Childs MB, et al. Medical costs of treating venous stasis ulcers: evidence from a retrospective cohort study. Vasc Med 1999;4(1):1–7.

60. Rice JB, Desai U, Cummings AK, et al. Burden of venous leg ulcers in the United States. J Med Econ 2014;17(5):347–56.

61. Vasquez MA, Rabe E, McLafferty RB, et al. Revision of the venous clinical severity score: venous outcomes consensus statement: special communication of the American Venous Forum Ad Hoc Outcomes Working Group. J Vasc Surg 2010;52(5): 1387–96.

62. Nicolaides AN. Investigation of chronic venous insufficiency: a consensus statement (France, March 5-9, 1997). Circulation 2000;102(20): E126–63.

63. Khilnani NM, Grassi CJ, Kundu S, et al. Multi-society consensus quality improvement guidelines for the treatment of lower-extremity superficial venous insufficiency with endovenous thermal ablation from the Society of Interventional Radiology, Cardiovascular Interventional Radiological Society of Europe, American College of Phlebology and Canadian Interventional Radiology Association. J Vasc Interv Radiol 2010;21(1): 14–31.

64. Bays RA, Healy DA, Atnip RG, et al. Validation of air plethysmography, photoplethysmography, and duplex ultrasonography in the evaluation of severe venous stasis. J Vasc Surg 1994;20(5):721–7.

65. Dauzat MM, Laroche JP, Charras C, et al. Real-time B-mode ultrasonography for better specificity in the noninvasive diagnosis of deep venous thrombosis. J Ultrasound Med 1986;5(11):625–31.

66. Shabani Varaki E, Gargiulo GD, Penkala S, et al. Peripheral vascular disease assessment in the lower limb: a review of current and emerging noninvasive diagnostic methods. Biomed Eng Online 2018;17(1):61.

67. DePopas E, Brown M. Varicose veins and lower extremity venous insufficiency. Semin Intervent Radiol 2018;35(1):56–61.

68. Wolpert LM, Rahmani O, Stein B, et al. Magnetic resonance venography in the diagnosis and management of May-Thurner syndrome. Vasc Endovascular Surg 2002;36(1):51–7.

69. Asciutto G, Mumme A, Marpe B, et al. MR venography in the detection of pelvic venous congestion. Eur J Vasc Endovasc Surg 2008;36(4):491–6.

70. Neglén P, Raju S. Intravascular ultrasound scan evaluation of the obstructed vein. J Vasc Surg 2002;35(4):694–700.

71. van den Bremer J, Moll FL. Historical overview of varicose vein surgery. Ann Vasc Surg 2010;24(3):426–32.

72. Zdravković D, Bilanović D, Randelović T, et al. [Friedrich Trendelenburg (1844 - 1924)–life and work]. Med Pregl 2006;59(3–4):183–5.

73. Royle J, Somjen GM. Varicose veins: hippocrates to Jerry Moore. ANZ J Surg 2007;77(12):1120–7.

74. Hettrick H. The science of compression therapy for chronic venous insufficiency edema. J Am Col Certif Wound Spec 2009;1(1):20–4.

75. O'Meara S, Cullum N, Nelson EA, et al. Compression for venous leg ulcers. Cochrane Database Syst Rev 2012;(11):CD000265.

76. Lerman M, Gaebler JA, Hoy S, et al. Health and economic benefits of advanced pneumatic compression devices in patients with phlebolymphedema. J Vasc Surg 2019;69(2):571–80.

77. Nelson EA, Mani R, Vowden K. Intermittent pneumatic compression for treating venous leg ulcers. Cochrane Database Syst Rev 2008;(2):CD001899.

78. Stacey MC, Jopp-Mckay AG, Rashid P, et al. The influence of dressings on venous ulcer healing–a randomised trial. Eur J Vasc Endovasc Surg 1997;13(2):174–9.

79. Luz BSR, Araujo CS, Atzingen DANCV, et al. Evaluating the effectiveness of the customized Unna boot when treating patients with venous ulcers. An Bras Dermatol 2013;88(1):41–9.

80. Ulloa JH. Micronized Purified Flavonoid Fraction (MPFF) for patients suffering from chronic venous disease: a review of new evidence. Adv Ther 2019;36(Suppl 1):20–5.

81. Katsenis K. Micronized purified flavonoid fraction (MPFF): a review of its pharmacological effects, therapeutic efficacy and benefits in the management of chronic venous insufficiency. Curr Vasc Pharmacol 2005;3(1):1–9.

82. Pittler MH, Ernst E. Horse chestnut seed extract for chronic venous insufficiency. Cochrane Database Syst Rev 2012;(11):CD003230.

83. Eckmann DM. Polidocanol for endovenous microfoam sclerosant therapy. Expert Opin Investig Drugs 2009;18(12):1919–27.

84. Alder G, Lees T. Foam sclerotherapy. Phlebology 2015;30(2 Suppl):18–23.

85. Rao J, Goldman MP. Stability of foam in sclerotherapy: differences between sodium tetradecyl sulfate and polidocanol and the type of connector used in the double-syringe system technique. Dermatol Surg 2005;31(1):19–22.

86. Forlee MV, Grouden M, Moore DJ, et al. Stroke after varicose vein foam injection sclerotherapy. J Vasc Surg 2006;43(1):162–4.

87. Rabe E, Pannier-Fischer F, Gerlach H, et al. Guidelines for sclerotherapy of varicose veins (ICD 10: I83.0, I83.1, I83.2, and I83.9). Dermatol Surg 2004;30(5):687–93 [discussion: 693].

88. Munavalli GS, Weiss RA. Complications of sclerotherapy. Semin Cutan Med Surg 2007;26(1):22–8.

89. Duffy DM. Small vessel sclerotherapy: an overview. Adv Dermatol 1988;3:221–42.

90. Samuel N, Carradice D, Wallace T, et al. Endovenous thermal ablation for healing venous ulcers and preventing recurrence. Cochrane Database Syst Rev 2013;(10):CD009494.

91. Barwell JR, Davies CE, Deacon J, et al. Comparison of surgery and compression with compression alone in chronic venous ulceration (ESCHAR study): randomised controlled trial. Lancet 2004; 363(9424):1854–9.

92. Howard DP, Howard A, Kothari A, et al. The role of superficial venous surgery in the management of venous ulcers: a systematic review. Eur J Vasc Endovasc Surg 2008;36(4):458–65.

93. Gohel MS, Heatley F, Liu X, et al. A randomized trial of early endovenous ablation in venous ulceration. N Engl J Med 2018;378(22):2105–14.

94. Sufian S, Arnez A, Labropoulos N, et al. Incidence, progression, and risk factors for endovenous heat-induced thrombosis after radiofrequency ablation. J Vasc Surg Venous Lymphat Disord 2013;1(2): 159–64.

95. Kabnick LS, Sadek M, Bjarnason H, et al. Classification and treatment of endothermal heat-induced thrombosis: recommendations from the American venous Forum and the Society for Vascular Surgery. J Vasc Surg Venous Lymphat Disord 2021; 9(1):6–22.

96. Rasmussen LH, Lawaetz M, Bjoern L, et al. Randomized clinical trial comparing endovenous laser ablation, radiofrequency ablation, foam sclerotherapy and surgical stripping for great saphenous varicose veins. Br J Surg 2011;98(8): 1079–87.

97. Tang TY, Rathnaweera HP, Kam JW, et al. Endovenous cyanoacrylate glue to treat varicose veins and chronic venous insufficiency-Experience gained from our first 100+ truncal venous ablations in a multi-ethnic Asian population using the Medtronic VenaSeal™ Closure System. Phlebology 2019; 34(8):543–51.

98. Kolluri R, Chung J, Kim S, et al. Network meta-analysis to compare VenaSeal with other superficial venous therapies for chronic venous insufficiency. J Vasc Surg Venous Lymphat Disord 2020;8(3): 472–81.e3.

99. Sermsathanasawadi N, Hanaroonsomboon P, Pruekprasert K, et al. Hypersensitivity reaction after cyanoacrylate closure of incompetent saphenous veins in patients with chronic venous disease: a retrospective study. J Vasc Surg Venous Lymphat Disord 2021;9(4):910–5.

100. Parsi K, Kang M, Yang A, et al. Granuloma formation following cyanoacrylate glue injection in

peripheral veins and arteriovenous malformation. Phlebology 2020;35(2):115–23.

101. Langridge BJ, Onida S, Weir J, et al. Cyanoacrylate glue embolisation for varicose veins - a novel complication. Phlebology 2020;35(7):520–3.

102. van Eekeren RRJP, Boersma D, Holewijn S, et al. Mechanochemical endovenous ablation versus RADiOfrequeNcy ablation in the treatment of primary great saphenous vein incompetence (MARADONA): study protocol for a randomized controlled trial. Trials 2014;15:121.

103. Elias S, Raines JK. Mechanochemical tumescentless endovenous ablation: final results of the initial clinical trial. Phlebology 2012;27(2):67–72.

104. Bishawi M, Bernstein R, Boter M, et al. Mechanochemical ablation in patients with chronic venous disease: a prospective multicenter report. Phlebology 2014;29(6):397–400.

105. van Eekeren RR, Boersma D, Elias S, et al. Endovenous mechanochemical ablation of great saphenous vein incompetence using the ClariVein device: a safety study. J Endovasc Ther 2011; 18(3):328–34.

106. Raju S. Treatment of iliac-caval outflow obstruction. Semin Vasc Surg 2015;28(1):47–53.

107. Lichtenberg MKW, de Graaf R, Stahlhoff WF, et al. Venovo venous stent in the treatment of non-thrombotic or post-thrombotic iliac vein lesions - short-term results from the Arnsberg venous registry. Vasa 2019; 48(2):175–80.

108. Razavi MK, Black S, Gagne P, et al. Pivotal study of endovenous stent placement for symptomatic iliofemoral venous obstruction. Circ Cardiovasc Interv 2019;12(12):e008268.

109. Shamimi-Noori SM, Clark TWI. Venous stents: current status and future directions. Tech Vasc Interv Radiol 2018;21(2):113–6.

110. Rasmussen L, Lawaetz M, Serup J, et al. Randomized clinical trial comparing endovenous laser ablation, radiofrequency ablation, foam sclerotherapy, and surgical stripping for great saphenous varicose veins with 3-year follow-up. J Vasc Surg Venous Lymphat Disord 2013;1(4):349–56.

111. Olivencia JA. Minimally invasive vein surgery: ambulatory phlebectomy. Tech Vasc Interv Radiol 2003;6(3):121–4.

112. Sadick NS, Wasser S. Combined endovascular laser plus ambulatory phlebectomy for the treatment of superficial venous incompetence: a 4-year perspective. J Cosmet Laser Ther 2007;9(1): 9–13.

113. Ricci S. Ambulatory phlebectomy. Principles and evolution of the method. Dermatol Surg 1998; 24(4):459–64.

Raynaud Phenomenon and Other Vasospastic Disorders

Ana I. Casanegra, MD, MS*, Roger F. Shepherd, MB BCh

KEYWORDS

- Raynaud syndrome • Primary Raynaud phenomenon • Secondary Raynaud phenomenon
- Acrocyanosis • Livedo reticularis • Pernio • Vasospastic disorders

KEY POINTS

- Primary vasospastic disorders are usually benign and require reassurance and conservative measures with avoidance of cold exposure.
- Some secondary vasospastic disorders may progress to digital ulceration and tissue loss. The prognosis depends on the underlying condition.
- The diagnosis is clinical, but laboratory testing, noninvasive testing, and imaging help to differentiate primary versus secondary vasospastic conditions.

INTRODUCTION

Raynaud syndrome and associated vasospastic disorders are commonly encountered in clinical cardiovascular practice. It is imperative for the clinician to understand the pathophysiology of vasospastic disorders and the recognize diverse presentations and natural history to appropriately manage these patients.

The term vasospasm indicates vasoconstriction of small blood vessels in the extremities, often precipitated by cold exposure. Primary (or idiopathic) vasospastic disorders implies that there is no underlying disease and consequently these patients often have a benign course; treatment focuses on control of symptoms. Secondary vasospastic disorders are associated with an underlying condition such as a connective tissue disease, atherosclerosis, vasculitis, drugs or toxins, or a hematologic disorder. These patients have an increased risk of tissue loss and digital ulcerations or gangrene; treatment should focus on the underlying condition. In this article, we review Raynaud syndrome, acrocyanosis, livedo reticularis, and pernio.

RAYNAUD SYNDROME
Introduction and Epidemiology

Acute episodic color changes in the digits were initially described by Maurice Raynaud, a French physician, in 1862. He presented a series of cases ranging from discoloration to gangrene of the digits.[1] Nowadays, the term "Raynaud syndrome" is used to describe episodic attacks of well-demarcated blanching or cyanosis of the digits on exposure to cold.[2]

In the literature, the terminology of Raynaud disease and Raynaud phenomenon can be misleading. To simplify this distinction, and avoid confusion, we refer to primary and secondary Raynaud syndrome throughout this review.

Primary Raynaud syndrome (historically known as Raynaud disease), indicates that there is no identifiable underlying cause and generally has a benign clinical course. Secondary Raynaud (historically Raynaud phenomenon) indicates vasospasm is a manifestation of an underlying condition. The prognosis depends on the underlying conditions and disease severity.

Vascular Medicine Division, Cardiovascular Department, Gonda Vascular Center, Mayo Clinic, 200 1st Street Southwest, Rochester, MN 55905, USA
* Corresponding author.
E-mail address: Casanegra.ana@mayo.edu

Cardiol Clin 39 (2021) 583–599
https://doi.org/10.1016/j.ccl.2021.06.010
0733-8651/21/© 2021 Elsevier Inc. All rights reserved.

The classic description of Raynaud syndrome consists of acute attacks of triphasic color changes of the digits brought on by exposure to cold or emotion, presenting with skin pallor owing to vasoconstriction, followed by cyanosis owing to deoxygenation, and finally rubor owing to hyperemia with release of vasoconstriction (**Figs. 1** and **2**).[3,4]

Raynaud syndrome is common in the general population with a prevalence estimated around 5%, and it is more common in females.[5] Although it can present at any age, it is more common in the second and third decades. A cold or damp climate is also associated with a higher prevalence of Raynaud syndrome, with a higher prevalence of 10% to 16%, and up to 37%, in colder or damp climates.[6]

Pathophysiology

The regulation of digital blood flow in normal individuals results from the interplay of the sympathetic nervous system, vascular tone, and hemorheological properties of the blood. Local humoral mediators such as nitric oxide and endothelin act on digital artery smooth muscle to maintain vessel tone and can induce vasodilation or vasoconstriction.

Although there are many theories as to the mechanism of vasospasm in Raynaud syndrome,

the exact cause is unknown. Theories include local vascular hyperreactivity, increased sympathetic nervous system activity, increased sensitivity of alpha 2 receptors to noradrenaline, increases in vasoconstrictor substances including thromboxane A2 from activated platelets, and increased production of endothelin-I from vascular endothelial cells. In a warm environment, digital blood flow in patients with Raynaud syndrome is similar to those without Raynaud syndrome; however, the flow at the fingertips diminishes with progressive environmental cooling.[7] Patient with Raynaud syndrome are felt to have an exaggerated vasoconstrictor response to cold. During cooling, the flow to the digits decreases, keeping enough capillary flow to ensure nutrition of the tissues, but decreasing heat loss through the hand and fingers.

The hands and fingers contain multiple arteriovenous anastomoses that can shunt the blood directly from the arterial to the venous circulation, bypassing the capillary bed.[8,9] The shunts open in a warm environment but close during cold exposure to maintain core body temperature.

In secondary Raynaud syndrome, baseline digital blood pressure is decreased as a result of underlying fixed occlusive disease or increased viscosity from hematologic conditions. In these patients, a normal sympathetic response to cold with vasoconstriction is more likely to induce closure of the blood vessel.

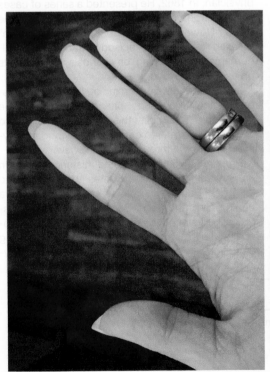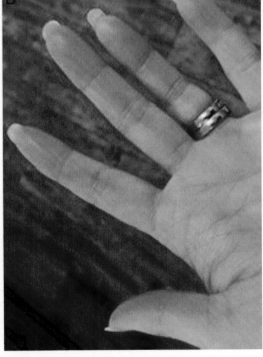

Fig. 1. Pallor (*A*) and rubor (*B*) during a Raynaud attack.

Step 1: Screening question

Are Your fingers unusually sensitive to cold?

Step 2: Assess color changes   **YES**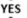

Occurrence of biphasic color changes during the vasospastic episodes (white and blue)

Step 3: Calculate disease score   **YES**

- Episodes are triggered by things other than cold (i.e. Emotional stressor)
- Episodes involve both hands, even if they involvement is asynchronous and/or asymmetric
- Episodes are accompanied by numbness and/ or paresthesia
- Observed color changes are often characterized by a well demarcated border between affected and unaffected skin
- Patient provided photographs strongly support a diagnosis of Raynaud's syndrome
- Episodes sometimes occur at other body sites (e.g. nose, ears, feet, areola)
- Occurrence of triphasic color changes during the vasospastic episodes (white, blue, red)

If 3 or more criteria from step 3 are met, the the patient has Raynaud's syndrome

Primary Raynaud's: 3 step criteria AND

Physical examination is negative for findings of secondary causes No history of existing connective tissue disease Normal capillaroscopy Negative or low titer ANA

Fig. 2. Diagnostic criteria for Raynaud syndrome and for primary Raynaud syndrome. ANA, antinuclear antibody. (*Adapted from* Maverakis E, Patel F, Kronenberg DG, et al. International consensus criteria for the diagnosis of Raynaud's phenomenon. *J Autoimmun.* 2014;48-49:60-65.)

Drugs can cause Raynaud syndrome through different mechanisms, including vasospasm, direct toxicity, endothelial damage, and other unclear mechanisms.

Primary Raynaud Syndrome

Primary Raynaud syndrome has a female predominance (females 9:1) with a usual onset in the second or third decades.[10] It is uncommon to develop symptoms after the age of 40 years.[4,10–12] There is a familial association in first-degree relatives, but a genetic culprit has not been identified.[5,10,13] Even though symptoms can be bothersome, this condition is benign condition because tissue loss and digital ulceration do not occur. Most patients remain stable with conservative or pharmacologic therapies.

Raynaud syndrome may affect 1 or 2 fingers initially, but eventually, most fingers of both hands are involved. The thumbs are often spared. The toes are commonly involved, and rarely the ears, nose, and areolar tissue are affected.[3,4,14,15]

There is an association with other vasospastic conditions, such as migraine headaches and Prinzmetal variant angina, suggesting a common background.[5,16] The likelihood of developing a connective tissue disease during follow-up is low (2.7 per 100 person-years), and patients can be reassured if the basic testing is negative (**Fig. 3**).[17]

Secondary Raynaud Syndrome

Any pathology causing decreased arterial pressure to the digits (eg, occlusion, compression, inflammation) can present with Raynaud syndrome. The 2 most common disorders are connective tissue diseases and atherosclerosis (**Box 1**, **Fig. 4**). The severity, frequency, and intensity of vasospastic attacks are worse in these patients and they may lead to digital ulceration, gangrene, and tissue loss (**Fig. 5**). The onset of symptoms is usually after the age of 50 years. The presence of red flags, such as nonsymmetric involvement, digital ulceration, and cardiovascular risk factors, should raise the suspicion for secondary Raynaud syndrome (see **Fig. 3**, red flag box).

Connective tissue disease

Raynaud phenomena can be associated with most connective tissue diseases, most commonly scleroderma and mixed connective tissue disease (see **Box 1**, **Fig. 6**).[18–22] It can also be the initial presentation, predating the diagnosis of the connective tissue disease.[18,19]

The majority of patients with systemic sclerosis (80%–95%) develop Raynaud syndrome, and in many cases Raynaud syndrome predates the diagnosis of a connective tissue disease.[18,19] The presence of "puffy fingers," telangiectasia and positive antinuclear antibodies, should raise the concern for early scleroderma.[18]

Arterial occlusive disease

Arterial stenosis proximal to the hand can decrease downstream digital intravascular pressure. A normal physiologic vasoconstrictor response to cold exposure in this case could precipitate temporary digital artery occlusion owing to a decrease in transmural distending forces and trigger an attack of Raynaud syndrome. The most prevalent underlying arterial disease is atherosclerosis. Less likely causes include arterial embolization.

Thromboangitis obliterans (Buerger's disease) is an inflammatory disease that commonly presents with distal ischemia of the fingers and toes. Raynaud syndrome is common in up to 40% of patients. Patients are usually younger than 45 years of age and all have a history of tobacco use.[23]

Drugs and toxins

Beta-blocker use was the most common reason for secondary Raynaud syndrome in 34.2% of patients.[24] Beta-blockers are not contraindicated in patients with Raynaud syndrome and can be prescribed if clinically indicated (eg, for coronary disease or hypertension).[25]

Methylphenidate and dextroamphetamine, stimulants used for the treatment of attention deficit hyperactivity disorder, have been associated with Raynaud syndrome.[26] High doses of ergot derivatives, used to treat migraine, cause vasospasm and, in rare cases, digital ischemia. Chemotherapeutic agents associated with Raynaud include bleomycin, vinblastine, carboplatin, and gemcitabine.[27]

Hematologic disorders

Raynaud syndrome may be associated with hyperviscosity syndromes and other hematologic disorders.[28] Primary or secondary cold agglutinin disease can present with Raynaud syndrome or acrocyanosis. Up to 91% of the patients with primary cold agglutinin disease have Raynaud syndrome.[29] Cryoglobulinemia is characterized by the presence of immunoglobulins that precipitate at cold temperature and dissolve on rewarming. It can manifest as Raynaud syndrome, acrocyanosis, and rarely cutaneous ulcers and gangrene. In these patients, Raynaud syndrome may involve the ears, lips, and tip of the nose.[30]

Miscellaneous causes

Nerve involvement in compression syndromes such as carpal tunnel syndrome or thoracic outlet

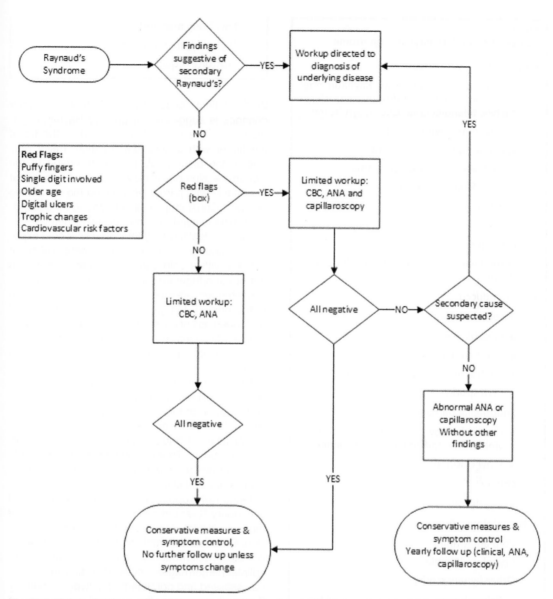

Fig. 3. Initial evaluation and follow-up in patients with Raynaud syndrome. ANA, antinuclear antibody; CBC, complete blood count.

syndrome rarely can present with Raynaud syndrome. In thoracic outlet syndrome, an embolic syndrome from a proximal subclavian aneurysm should be ruled out. Traumatic injuries to the hand and fingers in workers that operate vibrating machinery can cause hand–arm vibration syndrome in the dominant hand. It may be accompanied by neurologic symptoms such as tingling or paresthesia.[31]

Diagnosis

History and physical examination

Raynaud syndrome is a clinical diagnosis based on color changes of the fingers. It is rare to see

episodes of vasospasm in the office or in the vascular laboratory; pictures provided by patients can be helpful.

A thorough medical history and physical examination are key to guide the evaluation and management of Raynaud syndrome and help make the distinction between primary versus secondary Raynaud syndrome. An international consensus proposed a 3-step approach for the diagnosis of Raynaud syndrome (see **Fig. 2**).[3]

Most patients with Raynaud syndrome report biphasic color changes with pallor and cyanosis alone. Typical triphasic color changes are not required to make the diagnosis (see **Figs. 1** and

Box 1
Causes of secondary Raynaud syndrome

- Connective tissue disease
  - Systemic sclerosis/calcinosis, Raynaud phenomenon, esophageal dysfunction, sclerodactyly, telangiectasia (CREST) syndrome
  - Mixed connective tissue disease
  - Systemic lupus erythematous
  - Dermatomyositis or polymyositis
  - Primary Sjogren syndrome
- Arterial occlusive disease
  - Atherosclerosis
  - Arterial emboli
  - Thromboangeitis obliterans (Buerger's disease)
- Drug induced
  - Vasoconstrictors
    - Beta-blockers
    - Ergot alkaloids
    - Central nervous system stimulants
    - Cyclosporin
  - Endothelial damage
    - Chemotherapy agents: bleomycin, vinblastine, carboplatin, gemcitabine
    - Vinyl chloride
  - Other
    - Interferon
- Hematologic disorders
  - Cold agglutinins
  - Cryoglobulinemia
  - Other hyperviscosity
    - Polycythemia vera, hyperglobulinemia, HIV infection
    - Occupational arterial disease
- Miscellaneous
  - Nerve involvement
    - Carpal tunnel syndrome
    - Neurogenic thoracic outlet syndrome
  - Traumatic
    - Hand–arm vibration syndrome
- Endocrine
  - Hypothyroidism
  - Pheochromocytoma
  - Paraneoplastic

- Low body mass index
- Digital injury sequelae
- Frostbite sequelae

2).[3,4] Patient descriptions of triphasic color changes is suggestive of primary Raynaud syndrome.[4,12] The color changes start at the tip of the finger with a clear demarcation. Pallor may involve the distal phalanx or can extend to the webspace. Numbness may be present throughout the attack, with paresthesia during the rewarming phase.[14] Constant pain is concerning for secondary Raynaud syndrome and digital ischemia.

The principal trigger for the attacks is cold exposure, including minor changes in temperature or contact with a cold surface such as taking food out of the refrigerator or immersion in cold water. Other triggers are emotional stress (more common in the primary form), medications, vibration, and prolonged use of the digits.[4,24] It is important to review medications (including over-the-counter supplements), occupation, hobbies, and history of trauma.

The vascular examination should include bilateral brachial blood pressure, palpation of all pulses in the upper and lower extremities, Allen's test to ascertain patency of the radial and ulnar circulation in the hand, and auscultation over the large arteries for bruits. Thoracic outlet maneuvers should be performed to detect dynamic arterial compression. A detailed skin examination should focus on detection of trophic skin changes suggestive of secondary Raynaud syndrome, such as pitting of the nails, digital ulcerations, and thickening of the skin. Other dermatologic findings such as telangiectasias, sclerodactyly, dactylitis, malar rash, splinter hemorrhages, and livedo reticularis should be assessed and documented actively. In primary Raynaud syndrome, the physical examination is normal outside of the attacks. Fingers and toes, however, may be cold to the touch.

Laboratory studies

Laboratory testing is indicated if there is suspicion for secondary Raynaud and to risk stratify the patient for progression to a connective tissue disease. A blood count, urinalysis, and laboratory tests for renal function, thyroid function, antinuclear antibody, and inflammatory markers are a reasonable initial and cost-effective measures to detect secondary Raynaud syndrome. If the antinuclear antibody is positive, extractable nuclear antigen antibodies is the recommended next test.[14,32] Other autoantibodies may be indicated based on clinical presentation (see **Fig. 6**).

Secondary Raynaud's diagnosis

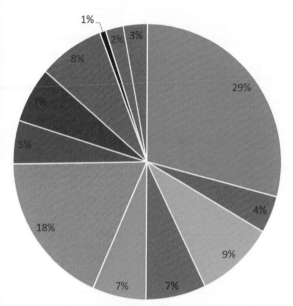

- 1%
- 2%
- 3%
- 8%
- 7%
- 5%
- 18%
- 7%
- 7%
- 9%
- 4%
- 29%

- ■ Scleroderma
- ■ MCTD
- ■ Undifferentiated CTD
- ■ SLE
- ■ Vasculitis
- ■ Atherosclerosis
- ■ Thromboangiitis obliterans
- ■ Hypothenar Hammer synd
- ■ Thoracic outlet
- ■ Amyloid
- ■ Chemotherapy
- ■ Malignancy

Fig. 4. Diagnosis of patients with secondary Raynaud. Mayo Clinic, Casanegra and Shepherd, unpublished data, 2021. CTD, connective tissue disease; MCTD, mixed connective tissue disease; SLE, systemic lupus erythematosus.

The presence of autoantibodies commonly found in systemic sclerosis and abnormal capillaroscopy increase the likelihood of systemic sclerosis or future development of systemic sclerosis; their absence is associated with a negative predictive value of 98%.[33]

Noninvasive vascular laboratory testing

Vascular laboratory tests are not used to make a diagnosis of Raynaud syndrome, but can help to differentiate between fixed occlusive disease and reversible vasospasm and help to guide the differential diagnosis.

Segmental pressure measurements and continuous wave Doppler tests These tests help to screen for proximal large vessel occlusive disease. A difference of more than 20 mm Hg between right and left brachial arteries, brachial-forearm systolic pressure gradient greater than 30 mm Hg, or

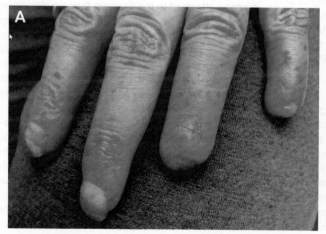

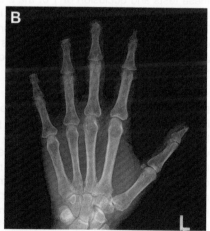

Fig. 5. Calcinosis, Raynaud phenomenon, esophageal dysfunction, sclerodactyly, telangiectasia (CREST) syndrome with telangiectasias, digital ulcers, and tissue loss (*A*), and acrolysis (*B*).

Condition	Symptoms	Associated antibody
Systemic sclerosis	Progressive fibrosis of the skin (scleroderma), "puffy fingers", arthralgias, telangiectasias, interstitial lung disease. Raynaud's syndrome (80–95%) CREST syndrome (Calcinosis, Raynaud's, Esophageal dysmotility, Sclerodactyly and Telangiectasia)	ANA, Anti topoisomerase I, anti centromere, anti RNA polymerase III
Mixed connective tissue disease	Myalgias, arthralgias, polymyositis, fever Raynaud's syndrome (93–100%)	ANA, Anti U1RNP
Systemic Lupus erythematous	Arthritis, cutaneous rash, thrombocytopenia, renal disease, vasculitis, Raynaud's syndrome (30–50%),	ANA, Anti-double-stranded DNA (anti-dsDNA)
Dermatomyositis /polymyositis	Muscle weakness, interstitial lung disease, skin rash Raynaud's syndrome	Anti-Ro, anti-La, anti-Sm, anti-ribonucleoprotein
Primary Sjoegren's syndrome	Ocular and oral dryness Raynaud's syndrome (10–50%)	ANA, Anti Ro/SS-A, anti La/SS-B

Fig. 6. Connective tissue diseases that can present with Raynaud syndrome. ANA, antinuclear antibody.

abnormal Doppler waveforms (monophasic or biphasic) are findings that should raise concern for proximal occlusive disease. The clinician should consider further imaging to evaluate these findings.

Digital systolic blood pressure Small digital cuffs wrapped around the proximal phalanx can measure systolic blood pressure and arterial perfusion can be qualitatively assessed with photoplethysmography, strain–gauge plethysmography, pulse volume recordings, or laser Doppler measurements.[34,35] Temperature may affect the results of these tests and occlusion of 1 of the 2 digital arteries can be missed if the other artery is patent. The digital pressure is commonly reported as a digital brachial index, and values of less than 0.8 are abnormal; however, criteria may differ between laboratories.

Photoplethysmography Photoplethysmography is performed with a light source and a photodetector affixed to the distal phalanx to estimate volumetric changes in the evaluated area. Changes in volume are assumed to represent changes in blood flow. Patients with primary Raynaud syndrome have a homogeneous pattern of normal waveforms.[36] Photoplethysmography has a sensitivity of 92% and specificity of 42% to predict occlusion of digital arteries compared with angiography.[36]

Digital temperature and thermography There is a correlation between blood flow and temperature at the fingers; thus, temperature can be used as a surrogate.[37] Temperatures are measured at the fingertip with constant room temperature to avoid variations.[38] Patients with Raynaud syndrome will present with low temperatures at baseline and will take longer to return to baseline after a cold challenge.[39] Protocols are not standardized, making comparisons challenging.[40]

Laser Doppler flowmetry, laser Doppler imaging, and laser speckle contrast imaging Laser Doppler flowmetry measures real-time skin blood flow with a probe attached to the fingertip through detection of a Doppler shift of a laser reflecting on moving structures like the erythrocytes.[41] It is expressed as an arbitrary unit. Laser Doppler imaging relies on the same phenomenon as Laser Doppler flowmetry, but evaluates a larger area without direct contact, at the expense of longer acquisition time and low resolution.[41]

Laser Doppler spectral contrast imaging analyzes interference of scattered light in a pattern called speckle. The fluctuations of the speckle pattern can be analyzed to obtain information about blood flow. It allows real-time, contactless imaging and has a short acquisition time.[41]

Because none of these methods can quantify flow, they are commonly used for comparison between fingers in association with thermal challenges.[38,41,42] Laser Doppler flowmetry at baseline and after heat provocation had a high sensitivity and specificity to detect fixed occlusive disease when compared with angiography (**Fig. 7**).[42]

Imaging

Duplex ultrasound examination, magnetic resonance angiography, and contrast-enhanced computed tomographic angiography are used commonly to evaluate the large vessels of the upper extremity and can help determine other coexisting conditions. Catheter-based angiography may be indicated in select patients, such as those with a clinical concern for distal embolization or thromboangitis obliterans, because it has excellent resolution of the digital arteries when performed by experienced operators.

Nailfold capillaroscopy

The capillaries of the nail fold easily are visualized parallel to the skin surface. Systemic sclerosis and other connective tissue diseases are known to affect them in distinctive patterns, and can aid in the early detection of disease, be used to confirm a diagnosis, or predict progression to a connective tissue disease (**Fig. 8**).[43] The gold standard is video capillaroscopy, which has a high resolution and allows for the measurement of capillary size and density. Other methods include stereo microscope, dermatoscope, ophthalmoscope, and USB microscope. They are less expensive and portable, at the cost of lower magnification and image quality.[43]

Therapeutic Options

There is no cure for primary Raynaud syndrome and therefore therapies are directed at alleviating symptoms by decreasing the frequency and severity of the attacks. Most patients with primary Raynaud syndrome have mild symptoms that can be controlled with protection from cold and avoidance of triggers.

In contrast, patients with secondary Raynaud syndrome can develop digital ischemia and ulceration. Strategies to improve blood flow based on vasodilator medications have limited effect in those with fixed occlusive disease. In addition to symptom management, the treatment plan needs to address the underlying disease with referral to an appropriate specialist.

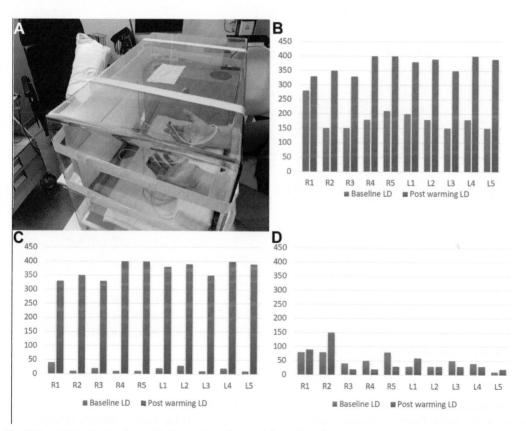

Fig. 7. Laser Doppler testing with thermal challenge. (*A*) Hot box fingers warming. (*B*) Normal subject. (*C*) Vasospasm. (*D*) Fixed occlusive disease.

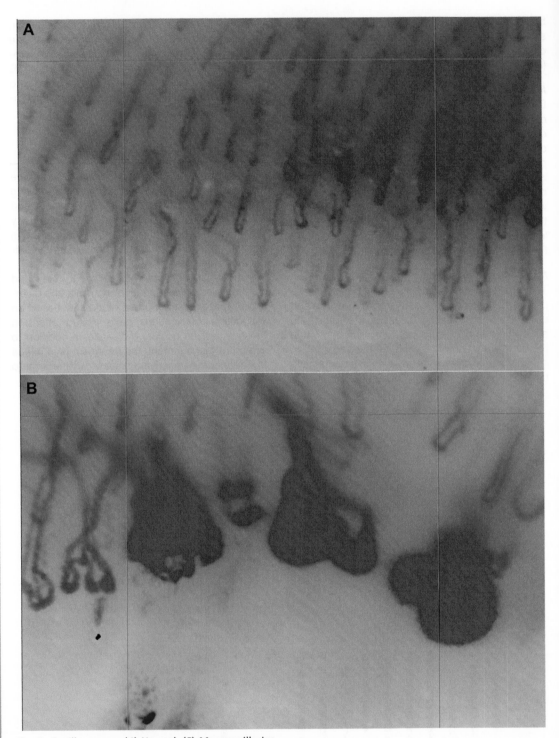

Fig. 8. Capillaroscopy. (*A*) Normal. (*B*) Megacapillaries.

Nonpharmacologic modalities

Preventive measures Patients should avoid cold exposure and dress warmly. The whole body needs to be warm to avoid vasoconstriction of the extremities to conserve body heat.[44] Hand warmers could be used in primary Raynaud syndrome, but are discouraged in patients with secondary Raynaud syndrome owing to the concern of inadvertent burns.[44] Vasoconstrictors such as decongestants, weight loss pills, stimulants, and tobacco should be avoided.

Biofeedback and other complementary therapies
Biofeedback has been studied in several randomized trials with variable results. A meta-analysis was inconclusive owing to the heterogeneity of the studies.[45] Other alternative therapies evaluated with at least 1 positive study are acupuncture, herbal supplement of gingko biloba extract, and fish oil supplementation.[46]

Pharmacologic therapies
One-half of patients with Raynaud syndrome do not respond to any vasodilator medication.

Calcium channel blockers These agents are generally well-tolerated with limited side effects of lower extremity edema, headaches, flushing, and constipation.[47] In a systematic review including patients with either primary or secondary Raynaud syndrome, those taking nifedipine had fewer attacks per week and the attacks were shorter in duration.[48]

Dihydropyridine calcium channel blockers have the most potent vasodilator effect within this group. It is advised to start at a low dose and increase as tolerated, depending on symptoms. Nifedipine (long acting)[48] and amlodipine are the most common medication choices.[47] Diltiazem and verapamil have less of a vasodilator effect and should not be used for Raynaud.

Alpha adrenergic blockers Studies noted improvement in noninvasive testing and symptoms with alpha adrenergic blockers.[49] The most common side effect is postural hypotension, but individuals usually develop tolerance. Symptoms can be minimized by starting at a low dose at night and increasing every few days to a target dose, depending on symptoms. Doxazosin and terazosin have a longer half-life and offer daily dosing.[50]

Renin–angiotensin system inhibitors Activation of the renin–angiotensin system is not a primary cause of vasoconstriction in Raynaud syndrome; however, a few small studies have shown symptomatic benefit in patients treated with losartan[51] or captopril.[52] Angiotensin-converting enzyme inhibitors should be included in all patients with systemic sclerosis and hypertension to prevent a sclerodermal renal crisis.

Phosphodiesterase type 5 inhibitors A meta-analysis of phosphodiesterase type 5 inhibitors (sildenafil, tadalafil, and vardenafil), including predominantly secondary Raynaud syndrome owing to systemic sclerosis, showed a decrease in the frequency and duration of digital ischemic attacks.[53] Small studies report improved ulcer healing in patients with systemic sclerosis when treated with phosphodiesterase type 5 inhibitors.[54]

Endothelin antagonists Bosentan is an antagonist of the endothelin 1 receptor, and it is used for treatment of pulmonary hypertension. Studies on patients with systemic sclerosis have shown improvement in Raynaud attacks, improved healing of digital ulcers or reduction in the number of new ulcers.[55] Bosentan is contraindicated in pregnancy owing to malformations and fetal loss.

Prostaglandins Intravenous iloprost is recommended in Europe for the treatment of digital ulcers in systemic sclerosis when other treatments have failed, and for refractory Raynaud syndrome not responding to other therapies.[56] It is not approved in the United States.

Botulinum toxin Botulinum toxin can be administered via local injection in the digital web spaces near the digital arteries. The mechanism proposed for the effect includes the inhibition of sympathetic vasoconstriction, release of endothelin, and inhibition of sensory nerves.[57] The data on efficacy are limited to small studies. In patients with systemic sclerosis, symptoms improved with active treatment.[58] Owing to minimal side effects, it can be attempted before a sympathectomy in patients with refractory symptoms.

Topical therapies Topical nitrates may be better tolerated with lower incidence of side effects. A meta-analysis comparing topical nitrates with placebo favored the treatment arm, despite the challenge of having different compounds and vehicles.[59] Other medications that can be topically administered include calcium channel blockers and phosphodiesterase type 5 inhibitors.[60]

Other Therapies

Sympathectomy
Sympathectomy can be used to relieve ischemic pain in the upper extremities. It involves lysis of the sympathetic nerves at the neck, thorax, or digits.[61] The effects tend to be short lived in primary Raynaud syndrome, and more persistent in secondary Raynaud syndrome. Distal sympathectomy (hand and digital) seems to have enduring effects, depending on the surgical technique and extension of the procedure. Owing to the invasive nature of the procedure, it should be considered a last resort in patients with tissue loss who have failed medical therapy.[62]

Box 2
Causes of secondary acrocyanosis

- Autoimmune diseases
    - Antiphospholipid syndrome
    - Connective tissue disease
- Hematologic disorders
    - Cold agglutinin
    - Cryoglobulinemia
    - Myeloproliferaitive disorders
- Neurologic disorders
    - Paraplegia
    - Multiple sclerosis
    - Postural orthostatic tachycardia syndrome
    - Orthostatic intolerance
- Starvation and eating disorders
- Malignancy
- Infection
- Inherited metabolic disorders
- Drug induced
    - Vasoconstrictors
    - Interferon
    - Chemotherapy
    - Biological agents

Other therapies for refractory ulcers

Hyperbaric oxygen therapy and intermittent pneumatic compression can be used as adjunctive therapies for refractory digital ulcers in patients with Raynaud syndrome.[63,64]

ACROCYANOSIS

Acrocyanosis is the symmetric painless discoloration of distal parts of the body (usually hands and feet), aggravated by cold or dependency.[65] The prevalence is unknown because there are no strict definition criteria. Pathophysiology has not been well-established, but may be related to autonomic function abnormality.

As with Raynaud, acrocyanosis may be divided into primary (idiopathic) or secondary. Primary acrocyanosis is a generally benign condition requiring no specific treatment, more commonly affecting women in the second and third decades. Secondary acrocyanosis is a manifestation of other diseases. Prognosis depends on the underlying disorder (**Box 2**).[65,66]

The most common finding is persistent, symmetric, painless purple or cyanotic discoloration of hands and feet that worsens with dependency and improves with elevation.[65] It can be associated with hyperhidrosis of the affected areas and with other vasospastic disorders.[65] Testing might be indicated to rule out secondary causes. Delayed age of onset, asymmetry, pain, and ulcerations are suggestive of secondary acrocyanosis.

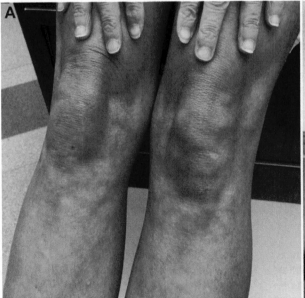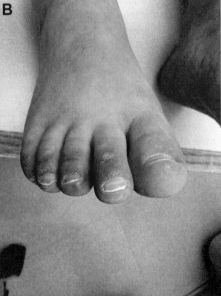

Fig. 9. (*A*) Primary livedo reticularis. (*B*) Pernio.

There is no effective treatment for primary acro-cyanosis, although multiple agents, including cal-cium channel blockers, beta-blockers, and nicotinic acid derivatives have been investigated. For secondary acrocyanosis, treatment should focus on the underlying disorder.

LIVEDO RETICULARIS

Livedo reticularis is a violaceous reticular discolor-ation of the skin involving more commonly the ex-tremities, but can affect other sites (**Fig. 9**). The peripheral venous plexuses of the skin become visible when there is venodilation or deoxygen-ation of the blood.

Livedo reticularis can be primary or secondary. There is a female predominance in the primary form. The discoloration of livedo reticularis can be transient or fixed. It is usually asymptomatic and does not require therapy. Avoiding cold expo-sure and vasoconstrictors may improve the appearance.[67]

Livedo racemosa describes an irregular red to violet branching discoloration of the skin; it is not blanchable and always represents an underlying occlusive or inflammatory pathology.[68]

Numerous pathologies are associated with livedo reticularis (**Box 3**) and include rheumato-logic disorders, hematologic disorders, neurologic syndromes, medications, infections, and malignancy.[69]

Cholesterol embolization from a more proximal artery can present with livedo reticularis. It can be provoked by catheter-based procedures and is frequently associated with acute renal failure.[70] Treatment is often supportive.

The diagnosis of livedo reticularis is based on clinical findings. A complete physical examina-tion and medical history should be obtained, along with a review of medications. Laboratory studies and other diagnostic tests should be guided by the findings in the history and phys-ical examination. A complete blood count with differential, antiphospholipid antibodies, and autoantibodies testing is reasonable. In the rare instance, a skin biopsy may be indicated; it should include the reticular dermis of the blanched and discolored area.[71] A skin biopsy may reveal cholesterol clefts diagnostic of atheroembolism.

PERNIO

Pernio, or chilblains, is an inflammatory disorder presenting with discoloration and edema of the skin, most commonly involving fingers and toes, caused by exposure to cold, nonfreezing

---

> **Box 3**
> **Causes of secondary livedo reticularis**
>
> - Cholesterol embolization syndrome
> - Rheumatologic
>   - Connective tissue disease
>   - Systemic lupus erythematosus
>   - Dermatomyositis
>   - Antiphospholipid syndrome
>   - Vasculitis
> - Hematologic disorders
>   - Cold agglutinins
>   - Cryoglobulinemia
>   - Multiple myeloma
>   - Other hyperviscosity
>   - Polycythemia vera, hyperglobulinemia, HIV infection
> - Neurologic
>   - Sneddon syndrome
>   - Postural orthostatic tachycardia syndrome
>   - Reflex sympathetic dystrophy
>   - Multiple sclerosis
>   - Spinal cord injury
> - Drug induced
>   - Vasoconstrictors
>   - Interferon
> - Infectious
>   - Hepatitis C
>   - Mycoplasma pneumonia
>   - Coxiella
>   - Severe acute respiratory syndrome corona virus 2
>   - Meningococcemia
> - Malignancy

---

conditions (see **Fig. 9**B). The prevalence is un-known, because many patients may not seek medical attention. It can affect any age with a pre-dominance of young females.[72] Lesions tend to recur every winter and improve in the summer.

Primary pernio is most common. Secondary pernio can be found in association with connective tissue diseases, cold agglutinins, hyperviscosity syndrome, and infections.

The skin lesions are usually painful reddish to purple papules or plaques, occasionally nodules and vesicles, that appear 12 to 24 hours after

> **Box 4**
> **Diagnostic criteria for pernio**
>
> Major criteria
>
> - Localized erythema and swelling involving acral sites persistent for more than 24 hours
>
> Minor criteria
>
> - Onset and/or worsening in cooler months
> - Histopathologic findings of skin biopsy consistent with pernio and without finding supporting lupus erythematosus
> - Response to conservative treatments
>
> Diagnosis requires presence of the major criterion PLUS one minor criteria.
> *Adapted from* Cappel JA, Wetter DA. Clinical characteristics, etiologic associations, laboratory findings, treatment, and proposal of diagnostic criteria of pernio (chilblains) in a series of 104 patients at Mayo Clinic, 2000 to 2011. *Mayo Clin Proc.* 2014;89(2):207-215.

cold exposure. The lesions usually heal in 2 to 3 weeks; however, some patients present with chronic disease. Elderly patients or those with secondary pernio are more likely to have digital ulceration. Keeping the affected area warm and dry will suffice to improve most lesions. Vasodilators (calcium channel blockers or alpha blockers) can be used if conservative measures are not enough. Additional therapies directed to the underlying etiology should be implemented in secondary pernio.[72]

A detailed history and physical examination to evaluate for systemic associated conditions should guide laboratory studies and biopsy should be considered only in patients with suspected secondary pernio without diagnosis or worsening despite therapy. Clinical diagnostic criteria have been proposed (**Box 4**).[72]

SUMMARY

Vasospastic disorders including Raynaud syndrome, acrocyanosis, livedo reticularis, and pernio are commonly encountered in cardiovascular practice. Primary vasospastic disorders have a benign course and respond to conservative measures and vasodilators. Secondary vasospastic disorders, in contrast, may result in tissue loss and digital gangrene. We have reviewed common secondary causes, initial diagnosis and management of primary and secondary vasospastic disorders. Distinguishing between the 2 has important prognostic and therapeutic considerations.

CLINICS CARE POINTS

> - Primary vasospastic disorders are managed with reassurance and conservative measures such as avoidance of cold exposure. They have a benign course and do not result in ulcers or tissue loss.
> - Secondary vasospastic disorders may result in tissue loss. The prognosis and management will depend on the underlying disease.
> - CBC, ANA and capillaroscopy are the initial workup for Raynaud's phenomenon. Other tests will be indicated based on the history and physical, and laboratory findings.
> - Patients need to be well protected from cold, not just at the affected areas but it's important to maintain adequate core temperature.
> - If conservative measures are not enough to control the symptoms, vasodilators can be initiated.

DISCLOSURE

The authors have nothing to disclose.

REFERENCES

1. Raynaud M. On local asphyxia and symmetrical gangrene of the extremities. London (UK): The New Sydenham Society; 1888.
2. Coffman JD. Raynaud's phenomenon. Oxford (UK): Oxford University Press; 1989.
3. Maverakis E, Patel F, Kronenberg DG, et al. International consensus criteria for the diagnosis of Raynaud's phenomenon. J Autoimmun 2014;48-49:60–5.
4. Gifford RW, Hines EA. Raynaud's disease among women and girls. Circulation 1957;16(6):1012–21.
5. Garner R, Kumari R, Lanyon P, et al. Prevalence, risk factors and associations of primary Raynaud's phenomenon: systematic review and meta-analysis of observational studies. BMJ Open 2015;5(3):e006389.
6. Maricq HR, Carpentier PH, Weinrich MC, et al. Geographic variation in the prevalence of Raynaud's phenomenon: a 5 region comparison. J Rheumatol 1997;24(5):879–89.
7. Greenfield ADM, Shepherd JT, Whelan RF. The loss of heat from the hands and from the fingers immersed in cold water. J Physiol 1951;112(3–4):459–75.
8. Coffman JD. Total and nutritional blood flow in the finger. Clin Sci 1972;42(3):243–50.

9. Coffman JD, Cohen AS. Total and capillary fingertip blood flow in Raynaud's phenomenon. N Engl J Med 1971;285(5):259–63.

10. Planchon B, Pistorius MA, Beurrier P, et al. Primary Raynaud's phenomenon. Age of onset and pathogenesis in a prospective study of 424 patients. Angiology 1994;45(8):677–86.

11. Pavlov-Dolijanovic S, Damjanov NS, Vujasinovic Stupar NZ, et al. Late appearance and exacerbation of primary Raynaud's phenomenon attacks can predict future development of connective tissue disease: a retrospective chart review of 3,035 patients. Rheumatol Int 2013;33(4):921–6.

12. Wollersheim H, Thien T. The diagnostic value of clinical signs and symptoms in patients with Raynaud's phenomenon. A cross-sectional study. Neth J Med 1990;37(5–6):171–82.

13. Freedman RR, Mayes MD. Familial aggregation of primary Raynaud's disease. Arthritis Rheum 1996; 39(7):1189–91.

14. Belch J, Carlizza A, Carpentier PH, et al. ESVM guidelines - the diagnosis and management of Raynaud's phenomenon. VASA Z Gefasskrankheiten 2017;46(6):413–23.

15. Chikura B, Moore T, Manning J, et al. Thumb involvement in Raynaud's phenomenon as an indicator of underlying connective tissue disease. J Rheumatol 2010;37(4):783–6.

16. Miller D, Waters DD, Warnica W, et al. Is variant angina the coronary manifestation of a generalized vasospastic disorder? N Engl J Med 1981;304(13): 763–6.

17. Ingegnoli F, Ughi N, Crotti C, et al. Outcomes, rates and predictors of transition of isolated Raynaud's phenomenon: a systematic review and meta-analysis. Swiss Med Wkly 2017;147:w14506.

18. Minier T, Guiducci S, Bellando-Randone S, et al. Preliminary analysis of the very early diagnosis of systemic sclerosis (VEDOSS) EUSTAR multicentre study: evidence for puffy fingers as a pivotal sign for suspicion of systemic sclerosis. Ann Rheum Dis 2014;73(12):2087–93.

19. Pearson DR, Werth VP, Pappas-Taffer L. Systemic sclerosis: current concepts of skin and systemic manifestations. Clin Dermatol 2018;36(4):459–74.

20. van den Hoogen F, Khanna D, Fransen J, et al. 2013 classification criteria for systemic sclerosis: an American College of Rheumatology/European League against Rheumatism collaborative initiative. Arthritis Rheum 2013;65(11):2737–47.

21. Gunnarsson R, Hetlevik SO, Lilleby V, et al. Mixed connective tissue disease. Best Pract Res Clin Rheumatol 2016;30(1):95–111.

22. Baldini C, Pepe P, Quartuccio L, et al. Primary Sjogren's syndrome as a multi-organ disease: impact of the serological profile on the clinical presentation of the disease in a large cohort of Italian patients. Rheumatol Oxf Engl 2014;53(5): 839–44.

23. Olin JW. Thromboangiitis obliterans (Buerger's disease). N Engl J Med 2000;343(12):864–9.

24. Brand FN, Larson MG, Kannel WB, et al. The occurrence of Raynaud's phenomenon in a general population: the Framingham Study. Vasc Med Lond Engl 1997;2(4):296–301.

25. Steiner JA, Cooper R, Gear JS, et al. Vascular symptoms in patients with primary Raynaud's phenomenon are not exacerbated by propranolol or labetalol. Br J Clin Pharmacol 1979;7(4):401–3.

26. Goldman W, Seltzer R, Reuman P. Association between treatment with central nervous system stimulants and Raynaud's syndrome in children: a retrospective case-control study of rheumatology patients. Arthritis Rheum 2008;58(2):563–6.

27. Campia U, Moslehi JJ, Amiri-Kordestani L, et al. Cardio-oncology: vascular and metabolic perspectives: a scientific statement from the American Heart Association. Circulation 2019;139(13):e579–602.

28. Gertz MA. Acute hyperviscosity: syndromes and management. Blood 2018;132(13):1379–85.

29. Berentsen S, Ulvestad E, Langholm R, et al. Primary chronic cold agglutinin disease: a population based clinical study of 86 patients. Haematologica 2006; 91(4):460–6.

30. Tedeschi A, Baratè C, Minola E, et al. Cryoglobulinemia. Blood Rev 2007;21(4):183–200.

31. Heaver C, Goonetilleke KS, Ferguson H, et al. Hand-arm vibration syndrome: a common occupational hazard in industrialized countries. J Hand Surg Eur Vol 2011;36(5):354–63.

32. Pistorius M-A, Carpentier P-H. Le groupe de travail « Microcirculation » de la Société française de médecine vasculaire. [Minimal work-up for Raynaud syndrome: a consensus report. Microcirculation Working Group of the French Vascular Medicine Society]. J Mal Vasc 2012;37(4):207–12.

33. Koenig M, Joyal F, Fritzler MJ, et al. Autoantibodies and microvascular damage are independent predictive factors for the progression of Raynaud's phenomenon to systemic sclerosis: a twenty-year prospective study of 586 patients, with validation of proposed criteria for early systemic sclerosis. Arthritis Rheum 2008;58(12):3902–12.

34. Blaise S, Constans J, Pellegrini L, et al. Optimizing finger systolic blood pressure measurements with laser Doppler: validation of the second phalanx site. Microvasc Res 2020;131:104029.

35. Nielsen PE, Bell G, Lassen NA. The measurement of digital systolic blood pressure by strain gauge technique. Scand J Clin Lab Invest 1972;29(4): 371–9.

36. Peller JS, Gabor GT, Porter JM, et al. Angiographic findings in mixed connective tissue disease. Correlation with fingernail capillary photomicroscopy and

digital photoplethysmography findings. Arthritis Rheum 1985;28(7):768–74.

37. Schlager O, Gschwandtner ME, Herberg K, et al. Correlation of infrared thermography and skin perfusion in Raynaud patients and in healthy controls. Microvasc Res 2010;80(1):54–7.

38. Wilkinson JD, Leggett SA, Marjanovic EJ, et al. A multicenter study of the validity and reliability of responses to hand cold challenge as measured by laser speckle contrast imaging and thermography: outcome measures for systemic sclerosis-related Raynaud's phenomenon. Arthritis Rheumatol 2018; 70(6):903–11.

39. Elstad M, Vanggaard L, Lossius AH, et al. Responses in acral and non-acral skin vasomotion and temperature during lowering of ambient temperature. J Therm Biol 2014;45:168–74.

40. Harada N. Cold-stress tests involving finger skin temperature measurement for evaluation of vascular disorders in hand-arm vibration syndrome: review of the literature. Int Arch Occup Environ Health 2002; 75(1–2):14–9.

41. Humeau-Heurtier A, Guerreschi E, Abraham P, et al. Relevance of laser Doppler and laser speckle techniques for assessing vascular function: state of the art and future trends. IEEE Trans Biomed Eng 2013;60(3):659–66.

42. Mahe G, Liedl DA, McCarter C, et al. Digital obstructive arterial disease can be detected by laser Doppler measurements with high sensitivity and specificity. J Vasc Surg 2014;59(4):1051–7.e1.

43. Cutolo M, Sulli A, Smith V. How to perform and interpret capillaroscopy. Best Pract Res Clin Rheumatol 2013;27(2):237–48.

44. Brajkovic D, Ducharme MB. Finger dexterity, skin temperature, and blood flow during auxiliary heating in the cold. J Appl Physiol (1985) 2003;95(2): 758–70.

45. Daniels J, Pauling JD, Eccleston C. Behaviour change interventions for the management of Raynaud's phenomenon: a systematic literature review. BMJ Open 2018;8(12):e024528.

46. Malenfant D, Catton M, Pope JE. The efficacy of complementary and alternative medicine in the treatment of Raynaud's phenomenon: a literature review and meta-analysis. Rheumatol Oxf Engl 2009; 48(7):791–5.

47. La Civita L, Pitaro N, Rossi M, et al. Amlodipine in the treatment of Raynaud's phenomenon. Br J Rheumatol 1993;32(6):524–5.

48. Rirash F, Tingey PC, Harding SE, et al. Calcium channel blockers for primary and secondary Raynaud's phenomenon [Systematic Review]. Cochrane Database Syst Rev 2017;12(12): CD000467.

49. Harding SE, Tingey PC, Pope J, et al. Prazosin for Raynaud's phenomenon in progressive systemic sclerosis. Cochrane Database Syst Rev 1998; 1998(2):CD000956. https://doi.org/10.1002/14651858.CD000956.

50. Paterna S, Pinto A, Arrostuto A, et al. [Raynaud's phenomenon: effects of terazosin]. Minerva Cardioangiol 1997;45(5):215–21.

51. Dziadzio M, Denton CP, Smith R, et al. Losartan therapy for Raynaud's phenomenon and scleroderma: clinical and biochemical findings in a fifteen-week, randomized, parallel-group, controlled trial. Arthritis Rheum 1999;42(12):2646–55.

52. Tosi S, Marchesoni A, Messina K, et al. Treatment of Raynaud's phenomenon with captopril. Drugs Exp Clin Res 1987;13(1):37–42.

53. Roustit M, Blaise S, Allanore Y, et al. Phosphodiesterase-5 inhibitors for the treatment of secondary Raynaud's phenomenon: systematic review and meta-analysis of randomised trials. Ann Rheum Dis 2013;72(10):1696–9.

54. Fries R, Shariat K, von Wilmowsky H, et al. Sildenafil in the treatment of Raynaud's phenomenon resistant to vasodilatory therapy. Circulation 2005;112(19): 2980–5.

55. Matucci-Cerinic M, Denton CP, Furst DE, et al. Bosentan treatment of digital ulcers related to systemic sclerosis: results from the RAPIDS-2 randomised, double-blind, placebo-controlled trial. Ann Rheum Dis 2011;70(1):32–8.

56. Ingegnoli F, Schioppo T, Allanore Y, et al. Practical suggestions on intravenous iloprost in Raynaud's phenomenon and digital ulcer secondary to systemic sclerosis: systematic literature review and expert consensus. Semin Arthritis Rheum 2019; 48(4):686–93.

57. Gallegos JE, Inglesby DC, Young ZT, et al. Botulinum toxin for the treatment of intractable Raynaud phenomenon. J Hand Surg 2021;46(1):54–9.

58. Motegi S-I, Uehara A, Yamada K, et al. Efficacy of botulinum toxin B injection for Raynaud's phenomenon and digital ulcers in patients with systemic sclerosis. Acta Derm Venereol 2017;97(7):843–50.

59. Curtiss P, Schwager Z, Cobos G, et al. A systematic review and meta-analysis of the effects of topical nitrates in the treatment of primary and secondary Raynaud's phenomenon. J Am Acad Dermatol 2018;78(6):1110–8.e3.

60. Wortsman X, Del Barrio-Díaz P, Meza-Romero R, et al. Nifedipine cream versus sildenafil cream for patients with secondary Raynaud phenomenon: a randomized, double-blind, controlled pilot study. J Am Acad Dermatol 2018;78(1):189–90.

61. Flatt AE. Digital artery sympathectomy. J Hand Surg 1980;5(6):550–6.

62. Coveliers HME, Hoexum F, Nederhoed JH, et al. Thoracic sympathectomy for digital ischemia: a summary of evidence. J Vasc Surg 2011;54(1): 273–7.

63. Sato T, Arai K, Ichioka S. Hyperbaric oxygen therapy for digital ulcers due to Raynaud's disease. Case Rep Plast Surg Hand Surg 2018;5(1):72–4.

64. Pfizenmaier DH, Kavros SJ, Liedl DA, et al. Use of intermittent pneumatic compression for treatment of upper extremity vascular ulcers. Angiology 2005;56(4):417–22.

65. Kurklinsky AK, Miller VM, Rooke TW. Acrocyanosis: the flying dutchman. Vasc Med Lond Engl 2011; 16(4):288–301.

66. Nousari HC, Kimyai-Asadi A, Anhalt GJ. Chronic idiopathic acrocyanosis. J Am Acad Dermatol 2001;45(6 Suppl):S207–8.

67. Gibbs MB, English JC, Zirwas MJ. Livedo reticularis: an update. J Am Acad Dermatol 2005;52(6): 1009–19.

68. Parsi K, Partsch H, Rabe E, et al. Reticulate eruptions: part 2. Historical perspectives, morphology, terminology and classification. Australas J Dermatol 2011;52(4):237–44.

69. Cervera R, Piette J-C, Font J, et al. Antiphospholipid syndrome: clinical and immunologic manifestations and patterns of disease expression in a cohort of 1,000 patients. Arthritis Rheum 2002;46(4):1019–27.

70. Fine MJ, Kapoor W, Falanga V. Cholesterol crystal embolization: a review of 221 cases in the English literature. Angiology 1987;38(10):769–84.

71. Wohlrab J, Fischer M, Wolter M, et al. Diagnostic impact and sensitivity of skin biopsies in Sneddon's syndrome. A report of 15 cases. Br J Dermatol 2001; 145(2):285–8.

72. Cappel JA, Wetter DA. Clinical characteristics, etiologic associations, laboratory findings, treatment, and proposal of diagnostic criteria of pernio (chilblains) in a series of 104 patients at Mayo Clinic, 2000 to 2011. Mayo Clin Proc 2014;89(2):207–15.

Moving?

Make sure your subscription moves with you!

To notify us of your new address, find your **Clinics Account Number** (located on your mailing label above your name), and contact customer service at:

Email: journalscustomerservice-usa@elsevier.com

800-654-2452 (subscribers in the U.S. & Canada)
314-447-8871 (subscribers outside of the U.S. & Canada)

Fax number: 314-447-8029

Elsevier Health Sciences Division
Subscription Customer Service
3251 Riverport Lane
Maryland Heights, MO 63043

*To ensure uninterrupted delivery of your subscription, please notify us at least 4 weeks in advance of move.

ELSEVIER

Printed and bound by CPI Group (UK) Ltd, Croydon, CR0 4YY

03/10/2024

01040306-0010